HERE'S THE PROBLEM . . .

On pregnancy, birth, and the newborn—

"Can you give us some tips on choosing the right doctor to take care if our expected baby?"

On night waking—

"Our six-month-old baby just won't go to sleep by himself. I know he's tired; he falls asleep in my arms. However, when I put him into his crib and try to tiptoe out of his room, he wakes up and screams. Help!"

Special concerns—

"I have recently begun coping with the role of a single parent following a divorce. I have custody of our two preschool children, but I am having trouble with discipline. Can you give me some tips?"

You'll find the solutions to these and 297 other questions in . . .

300 QUESTIONS NEW PARENTS ASK

WILLIAM SEARS, M.D., is a pediatrician in private practice in Pasadena, California, and an assistant professor of pediatrics at the University of Southern California. He is the author of eight books on child care and is a member of *Baby Talk* magazine's board of advisers. MARTHA SEARS, R.N., is a La Leche League Leader and a professional lactation consultant. Together William and Martha Sears host a weekly radio program, "Ask About Your Baby." They have seven children.

WILLIAM SEARS, M.D.
MARTHA SEARS, R.N.

3 0 0
QUESTIONS
NEW PARENTS
ASK

ABOUT PREGNANCY, CHILDBIRTH, AND INFANT & CHILD CARE

A PLUME BOOK

PLUME

Published by the Penguin Group
Penguin Books USA Inc., 375 Hudson Street,
New York, New York 10014, U.S.A.
Penguin Books Ltd, 27 Wrights Lane,
London W8 5TZ, England
Penguin Books Australia Ltd, Ringwood,
Victoria, Australia
Penguin Books Canada Ltd, 2801 John Street,
Markham, Ontario, Canada L3R 1B4
Penguin Books (N.Z.) Ltd, 182-190 Wairau Road,
Auckland 10, New Zealand

Penguin Books Ltd, Registered Offices:
Harmondsworth, Middlesex, England

First published by Plume, an imprint of New American Library,
a division of Penguin Books USA Inc.

First Printing, April, 1991
1 3 5 7 9 10 8 6 4 2

Copyright © Parenting Unlimited, Inc., 1991
All rights reserved

REGISTERED TRADEMARK—MARCA REGISTRADA

LIBRARY OF CONGRESS CATALOGING-IN-PUBLICATION DATA:

Sears, William, M.D
   300 questions new parents ask : about pregnancy, childbirth, and infant and
child care / William Sears, Martha Sears.
      p. cm.
   ISBN 0-452-26599-1
   1. Pregnancy—Miscellanea. 2. Childbirth—Miscellanea. 3. Infants—Care—
Miscellanea. 4. Child care—Miscellanea. I. Sears, Martha. II. Title. III. Title:
Three hundred questions new parents ask.
RG525.S3976 1991
618.2—dc20   90-20042
                                                                        CIP

Printed in the United States of America
Set in Century Expanded
Designed by Steven N. Stathakis

Publisher's note:
*The ideas, procedures, and suggestions contained in this book are not intended as
a substitute for consulting with your physician. All matters regarding your health
require medical supervision.*

BOOKS ARE AVAILABLE AT QUANTITY DISCOUNTS WHEN USED TO PROMOTE PROD-
UCTS OR SERVICES. FOR INFORMATION PLEASE WRITE TO PREMIUM MARKETING DIVI-
SION, PENGUIN BOOKS USA INC., 375 HUDSON STREET, NEW YORK, NEW YORK 10014.

We dedicate this book to our seven children, whose incessant questions have stimulated us to come up with many answers:

James
Robert
Peter
Hayden
Erin
Matthew
Stephen

Contents

INTRODUCTION

Over the past twenty years in our roles as pediatrician, father, mother, and nurse, we have been in the question-answering profession. Since 1985 we have hosted a weekly one-hour live call-in radio program called *Ask About Your Baby*. After responding to thousands of questions from concerned parents, we realized how deeply parents hunger for right answers. We also recognized that parents—because they deeply love their children, want to do the best, and fear they are not—are vulnerable to any child-rearing advice, good or bad, from a trusted person. Consequently, early in our Q & A career we developed a very committed sense of responsibility to the parents we counseled and the advice we gave. We practiced one of the basic medical principals—first do no harm. Children are too valuable and parents too vulnerable to be offered flippant, unresearched advice.

As our radio audience grew, our experience grew. We realized that most questions fall into the categories of feeding, sleeping, comforting, behavior, and illnesses. These categories form the basis of this book. Most of the questions in this book have been taken directly from transcripts of our radio program, together with questions from letters and office visits. These are real questions from real parents who want to do what is best for their children.

In addition to answering other parents' questions, during the parenting of our seven children we came up with our own questions which demanded answers. Nearly every question in this book we have personally asked in our family. We can truly say, "Yes, we understand, we've been there." Several times during our radio program we have apologized for audibly yawning from being tired. Yes, Dr. Bill's and Martha's babies wake up too! We are a busy family, as most of you are. We too have to juggle the spontaneous needs of children with the necessities of professional life-styles.

Our philosophy of baby care can be summed up in one word: *fit*. This tiny word economically describes our goal in writing this book. We want to help parents and babies fit together. This is why we discard rigid rules of parenting. We take the life-styles of the parents and the temperament of the baby and help you all fit together as a family. Fitting brings a sense of completeness to a relationship, a rightness that helps parents and baby enjoy each other. To help develop this fit, the answers in this book are geared toward a style of child care we call *attachment parenting*—a group of practical relationships with your child which, if practiced, result in what we believe are the three goals of parenting: to know your child, to help your child feel right (to develop a positive self-image), and to truly enjoy your child.

All the answers in this book are based upon a combination of scientific studies, our own personal experience, and the knowledge we have gained during the twenty-two years in our professional careers. Most of the answers contain two parts: First, we attempt to explain the reason why your baby acts the way he or she does; second, we offer practical advice to solve the individual problem. We sincerely hope that the advice offered in this book helps you and your baby bring out the best in each other.

1

PREGNANCY, BIRTH, AND THE NEWBORN

The material in this chapter is designed to help you prepare and care for your newborn. Most of the questions come from expectant parents whom we counseled before the birth of their child and from parents during the first few weeks after the birth of their child. In our office we call this *right start* counseling. Our goal for patients in our office and for the readers of this chapter is to help you develop a style of parenting in which you and your baby bring out the best in each other. Upon first glance you may consider the attachment style of parenting we foster in this chapter to be all giving, giving, giving. To a certain extent it is. Newborns are takers and parents are givers; that is a fact of parenting during the early months of a baby's life. However, there is another side to the parenting equation. The more the parents give to the baby, the more the baby gives back to the parents. This mutual giving leads to a mutual shaping of each other that helps all members of the family fit well together.

The style of parenting that we encourage in the opening chapter will help you organize your baby. One of a new

1

parent's most important functions is to help a baby become organized. Your newborn comes disorganized. His movements are random and jerky. Most of the cues he gives his parents seem purposeless and hard to decode. The style of parenting we encourage will help you read your baby's cues. Consequently, your baby becomes better organized, as does the whole family.

Much of the advice in these answers is designed to help parents develop a sensitivity toward their baby and the baby toward the parents. When parents and babies develop this mutual sensitivity they are well on the way to enjoying the ultimate goal of parenting—to enjoy each other.

1. *We are expecting our first baby and really want to do everything right. We have read a lot and attended expectant-parent classes. In short, this is a well-researched baby. Can you give us some tips on choosing among the various birthing options?*

Visit various hospitals and select a birthing option with which you feel most comfortable. We like your term "well-researched baby." We hear this term used often among today's parents, indicating that more and more of them are doing their homework. This movement has had an enrichening effect on the entire health care system.

The birthing option that we suggest for most parents is called the LDR room (older terms were ABC rooms or birthing rooms). The LDR room means that the mother labors, delivers, and recovers in the same room. The laboring couple is admitted to this room and does not leave the area until the mother and baby are discharged from the hospital. One distinct advantage of this birthing option is that mother and baby (and father) can stay together from the moment of birth to the time of discharge from the hospital. The LDR facility is more than just a room; it is a concept that gives the laboring couple the feeling that they are delivering in a home-like environment, but the attending medical personnel and necessary equipment are there in case a medical complication arises. Many mothers are intimidated by all the equipment in the traditional delivery room, which makes it look more like an operating room. In the LDR room, the same medical equipment is there but is hidden. The LDR is not just a fashionable trend—the concept began ten years ago. It is good medicine for both mother and baby. Since the mother does not have to be transported from a labor room to a delivery room to a recovery room, her labor is smoother. We have noticed that mothers in an LDR environment have less complicated labors. Their labors progress more smoothly because they have more space in which to move around. If your hospital does not offer an LDR option, you might wish to shop around. In time, all hospitals who hope to stay in the "baby business" will no doubt offer this option.

2. *We want to have an unmedicated labor and delivery, but we have heard many "war stories" about childbirth. Can you give us some tips on how we can increase our chances of having a natural childbirth?*

First of all, choose a hospital and a doctor who support your desires. Obtain good prenatal care and attend a good natural-childbirth class. Get tips from other mothers who have experienced natural childbirth. Most important select a birthing environment which encourages your labor to progress naturally—if possible, the LDR environment in a hospital or birthing center. During labor, go with the flow of your body. It is designed to tell you how to move and which position to assume during labor. A good childbirth class will prepare you to decode your body's signals. If your body tells you to move around, move around. If your body tells you to squat or even labor on all fours, then do it. Going with the flow of your body lessens the discomfort of labor, allows your labor to progress more efficiently, and lessens your chance of needing a cesarean section.

A word of advice about your desire to give birth to your baby naturally: When you enter the birthing environment, be flexible. While realizing that you are going to try to have your baby naturally, be prepared to shift gears if your doctor or birth attendant advises an alternative method of delivery because of a medical complication. If that happens, don't feel that you have failed. The main objective in childbirth is always a healthy baby and a healthy mother.

3. *We are expecting our first baby. Frankly, I am scared of all the technology that seems to be creeping into the childbirth experience. Can you put my mind at ease?*

Expectant couples are understandably confused about the benefits and risks of "technological" childbirth (involving medication, fetal monitoring, or induced labor) and natural childbirth (unmedicated). As a result, their confidence in their obstetrician or birth attendant is often undermined. Confidence in your doctor and your hospital is imperative to fully enjoying your childbirth experience. However, consumer questioning of technology is vital to keep technology in perspective, especially in such an important event as childbirth. If you have read something negative about your doctor's practices (e.g., medications, fetal monitoring), discuss your concerns with your obstetrician. Obstetrics is a medical specialty which is oriented toward minimizing the risks of childbirth. New obstetric technologies are designed to lower these risks, and have saved the lives of many mothers and babies. The choice between natural or technological childbirth should not be an either/or decision. We feel that obstetric care should respect parental intuition that technology be used appropriately rather than routinely. Neither the parents nor the baby should be deprived of the benefits of either method.

4. *We are expecting our second baby. My first delivery was very painful. I've heard that water birth is less painful. Is this true?*

Yes, laboring in warm water is less painful. Water birthing has been practiced in Russia and France for the past ten to twenty years. Only recently has this natural labor-saving device been used in the United States. Let us relay the experience from the obstetrical practice of a friend of ours, Dr. Michael Rosenthal. Between 1985 and 1990, at the Family Birthing Center of Upland, California, a thousand patients spent much of their labor in a Jacuzzi-type warm tub, the temperature of the water being around body temperature— 98 to 100 degrees. One half of these mothers went on to deliver their babies in water. The results were impressive. Not surprisingly, nearly all mothers reported less painful contractions and less back pain when immersed in water. Labors progressed more smoothly and the cesarean section rate was one third that of traditional hospitals. Only one mother (.1% overall) developed an easily treated infection (a much lower incidence than in traditional births) and there were no detrimental effects to the baby. The reason water works is simple: A relaxed mother has a relaxed uterus, which leads to a more normal labor. The buoyancy of water enables the mother to labor in the most comfortable position. The weightless feeling in water allows the mother to more easily support her body and deal with the contractions. Her muscles are less tense because they do not have to support her entire weight. As the mother relaxes, her stress hormones decrease and the natural birth-progressing hormones (oxytocin and endorphins) flow uninhibited. Birthing tubs are intended to be used to ease the pain and improve the progress of labor. Many women ultimately give birth in water because of their reluctance to emerge from it in spite of their impending delivery.

During my own labor with our seventh baby, Stephen, I experienced excruciating suprapubic pain. I went into the tub because I was having the type of pain that alerted me to do something to fix it. After trying the all-fours position and other comfort measures without relief, I realized I needed to try the water method. Water made it possible for me to relax and the pain melted away. For me, water labor was wonderful. When the birth was imminent, I got out of the tub and delivered on the bed. Then we saw the reason for the unusual pain—the baby's hand came out wedged alongside his head—a compound presentation.

We have studied the results of competent obstetricians who encourage water labor and water birthing in their practices. We conclude that over the next few years any hospital or birthing center who plans to stay in the baby business will be offering water labor to their obstetrical patients. In experienced hands, water labor is not just a passing fad but a growing reality. It is so simple! And it is simply good medicine, equally as effective as Demerol, with *none* of the side effects. Any method which eases discomfort and improves the health of the mother and baby during labor must be taken seriously. Between 1920 and 1980 obstetrics gradually excluded mothers from the central role in the birth process. In the 1980s and '90s water labor and water birthing is just one more step in giving childbirth back to women. (For an in-depth discussion of the benefits, techniques, and safety of water birthing, see the following reference: *Journal of Nurse—Midwifery*, Vol. 34, pp. 165–70, 1989.)

5. *We are considering a home birth, but are a little scared about this. Are home births safe?*

Before you decide, do your homework carefully. The American Academy of Obstetricians and Gynecologists (ACOG) has taken a wise position on home births, stating that *if couples are properly selected and the birth is properly attended*, home birthing may be as safe as hospital birthing. However, because of the possibility of unanticipated obstetrical complications, the best choice for most couples is a *home-like* birthing environment in an LDR room in a birthing center or hospital.

Following are some factors which might influence your decision about a possible home birth: If you have had previous uncomplicated deliveries, if your current pregnancy has been uncomplicated and if your doctor does not anticipate a pre-term delivery or unusual positioning (e.g., breech), if you have a normal prior obstetrical history, and, most important, if you have selected a qualified birth attendant with medical backup close by in case an unanticipated complication does arise, you may consider home birth. If you do choose a home birth attended by a qualified midwife, it is wise to also consult with an obstetrician in case specialized services are needed during and/or after delivery. Remember, childbirth is a very important event; for your expected baby, it is *the* most important event. Above all, you want to do everything possible to increase your chance of having a healthy baby and a healthy mother.

6. *Our first baby was delivered by cesarean section, and I would like to have my next baby vaginally. Is this possible?*

Yes, a vaginal birth after a cesarean is often possible. This birthing option is termed a VBAC—vaginal birth after cesarean. It used to be said, "Once a cesarean, always a cesarean," but this is no longer the case. Much depends on the reason for your previous section. If the reason was a problem occurring with that particular pregnancy or labor, such as breech presentation, fetal distress, or "failure to progress," then your chances of delivering your next baby vaginally are quite good. If, however, the reason for your previous section was cephalopelvic disproportion (your baby's head was too large to pass through your birth canal), then your chances of delivering your next baby vaginally may not be as good. During your next pregnancy, consult with your obstetrician concerning your chances of having a VBAC. The overall incidence of a successful VBAC is between sixty and seventy percent, but this figure varies considerably according to each mother's individual obstetrical history. Many mothers who birthed an eight-pound baby by cesarean go on to have VBAC babies of nine pounds or more. And each pregnany tends to widen your pelvis more. Some doctors report a seventy-five percent VBAC rate, so shop around for a doctor who truly understands VBAC management.

7. *I am now six months pregnant and have begun slight bleeding. Because of my past history of several miscarriages, my doctor advises me to stay in bed most of the time during the final three months. I resent being tied down like this, and am concerned my resentment may affect our baby. What is your opinion?*

Research into how the emotional state of the mother affects the emotional state of the fetus is still in its infancy, so to speak. Some researchers feel there is a close connection between a mother's emotional state and that of her pre-born baby, as if the same hormones which may be involved in your emotional state are transferred to your baby. Try the following: You have the advantage that many mothers do not—the opportunity for a long period of pre-birth bonding. During our seven pregnancies, we have noticed a natural nesting instinct that clicks in around the sixth or seventh month. It seems that a mother's mind and body are meant to slow down in the last three months of pregnancy and tune into the baby. Your medical condition actually forces you to do this. Rather than seeing this as being tied down, regard this time as an opportunity to enjoy the nesting instinct to its fullest. Many women do not have this luxury.

Talk and sing to your pre-born baby. Spend many hours each day simply thinking about your baby as you become truly aware of the person inside you. This "prenatal communication network" will enhance your bonding and communication with your baby *after* he or she is born. This is long-term bonding at its best.

8. *I am thirty-five and we are expecting our first baby. I know that having a baby at an older age increases the risk of having a baby with Down's syndrome. Should I worry?*

No. We feel that entirely too much anxiety is produced because misleading information is given to older parents who have babies. When the mother is between thirty-five and forty years of age, the risk of having a baby with

Down's syndrome is around one percent. This means that you have a ninety-nine percent chance of having a baby without Down's syndrome.

Legally, your doctor must inform you that there is a test called amniocentesis, which will detect whether or not your baby has Down's syndrome. This procedure is performed around the fourteenth or fifteenth week of pregnancy. You doctor inserts a needle through your abdomen into the amniotic cavity and obtains some amniotic fluid. This fluid is analyzed for abnormalities in fetal chromosomes, the sex of the baby, and specific chemical information that may suggest the presence of certain diseases. Amniocentesis is generally a safe procedure, but it is not without risks. The risk of injury to the fetus is usually less than one half of one percent when performed by experienced medical personnel. Because of the slight risk of injury to the fetus, many mothers elect not to have this procedure done. If you are extremely anxious about having a baby with Down's syndrome, spending an entire pregnancy with this anxiety is also not healthy for your pre-born baby. Some mothers choose this prenatal test to relieve their anxiety even though they would not consider having an abortion. There are newer tests (alpha fetal protein, followed by chorionic villus sampling if indicated) that can be performed even earlier in your pregnancy to detect the presence or absence of Down's syndrome even as early as ten weeks after conception. Chorionic villus sampling carries a higher risk to the developing baby, so we do not recommend it. Some mothers simply feel that the moment of birth is soon enough to become aware of any problem that could not be corrected while the baby is still *in utero*. Society, we feel, is gradually realizing that special babies truly *are* special babies. (See question 290 on caring for the Down's syndrome child).

9. *I'm thirty-nine years old and I feel my biological time clock is running out. I want to have another baby as soon as possible, but I'm afraid of delivering an abnormal baby because of my age. Should I be concerned?*

No! We feel that entirely too much unnecessary anxiety is caused by a fear of having babies in late thirties or early forties. Senior mothers often make more committed mothers since they have the benefit of more years of experience.

You should, however, avoid the pressure to have another baby "as soon as possible." Fertility experts have long noticed that often the pressure to conceive may actually prevent a couple from doing so. Many mothers are now delivering healthy babies in their early forties, so you should not feel unduly pressured by the mythical "biological time clock."

10. *Can you give us some tips on choosing the right doctor to take care of our expected baby?*

Look for two things: the doctor's competence and her communications abilities. Visit several doctors, either pediatricians or family doctors, the month before your baby is due. In our practice I like to meet with prospective parents before delivery.

Here is how to get the most out of your prenatal interview with the doctor:

• Make a written list of what you feel are the most important issues in parenting. Try to determine if your philosophies and those of the prospective doctor are in harmony.
• If you anticipate special needs, such as "I want to continue breastfeeding even though I'm returning to work. Can you help me with this?", communicate them.
• Obtain a list of the doctor's medical fees and office hours, and be sure that you are aware of which hospitals she is on the staff of and how easily she can be reached in emergencies.

Perhaps the best advice about an individual doctor's qualifications can be obtained by interviewing trusted friends who have used the particular doctor that you are considering.

The prenatal interview is also good for the doctor. It gives her an idea of what you really want and need as parents and also increases her respect for you. In our practice, we feel that if a parent has taken time to interview us wisely, this tells us something about their parenting priorities. Pediatrics is a specialty in which your doctor is going to grow in the knowledge of your child as your child grows. It is an investment of perhaps fifteen years or more. Make that investment wisely.

11. *Our baby is due any day now and we are going to buy a crib. Any suggestions on what to look for?*

First of all, we advise you not to invest a lot of money in a crib. Buy a used crib or borrow one temporarily to see if your baby will settle down readily in it. Many babies do, but others do not because they miss their mother. Their parents end up using the crib to collect toys and not for the baby to sleep in. Because many babies do not settle down well in cribs, you will probably have no trouble finding a used crib for sale. When you purchase a crib, here's what to look for:

1. Be sure the mattress fits the crib. Mattresses come in two basic constructions: coiled innerspring and foam rubber. Spring mattresses tend to be more expensive than foam. Good-quality mattresses have triple-laminated cloth or plastic covers which are waterproof and easily cleaned of stains and odors. If the cloth, plastic, or vinyl covering is too thin it will wear easily, tear easily, and may not be waterproof. Be sure the mattress cover is flame-retardant. Place the entire palm of your hand on the mattress. A good-quality mattress will have sufficient layers of felt and/or foam between the cover and the springs so that you cannot feel the springs. For babies under a year, a good-quality foam mattress around five inches thick will usually provide sufficient firmness so that you may not need the more expensive spring mattress.

2. Be sure the crib is adjustable so that it will accommodate your baby's changing height. Be sure the side rails can be easily removed so that the crib can be used as a side car next to your bed. Good quality cribs are equipped with steel stabilizing bars on both sides so that a railing can be removed while the stability of the crib is maintained.

3. Be sure the rail locks do not release too easily. You should have to lift the rail slightly before the lock releases so that the baby cannot do this alone.

4. Be sure that there are plastic teething strips attached to the top of the side rails to provide a chewing surface that prevents the baby from sinking his teeth into the wooden rail.

5. Raise and lower the side rails. Be sure there are noiseless bearings so that the crib does not squeak a lot when the side rails are raised and lowered. Your bedtime ritual can be defeated by raising a noisy crib rail just after you put a sleeping baby down.

6. Be sure the head and foot of your baby's crib have large, free-rolling casters which enable you to gently roll the crib back and forth to rock your baby to sleep.

7. The crib should be painted with a lead-free paint. Cribs manufactured after 1974 should have a sticker attesting to this. If they are manufactured before this date, inquire when they were painted and what type of paint was used. If there is no certainty that lead-free paint was used, don't buy the crib.

8. Crib slats should be no more than two and three eighths inches (six centimeters) apart to prevent your infant from slipping his body through the slats, hanging by the head and strangling. Bumper pads keep your baby's feet from dangling through the slats and allow him to push with his feet and propel himself around the crib. Metal hardware should be smooth and should not protrude into the crib. (See question 41 for additional crib-safety information.)

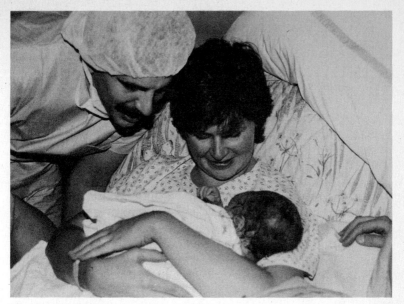

Bonding immediately after birth allows a new mother and father to get to know their baby.

12. *I've been warned our soon-to-be-born baby will not look like the clean, pink "picture book" baby in ads in magazines, but I'd like to have some idea what to expect. Can you tell me?*

Some writers have unfeelingly described the newly born baby as looking like a prize-fighter—after the fight. But as you examine your baby in the first hour after birth, you will probably find her very beautiful. Your baby's face and eyelids will appear puffy as a result of extra fluid accumulated beneath the skin. You will notice signs of your baby having had to squeeze a bit to enter the world. Her red face has areas of bluish-purple dotted with freckle spots from tiny broken blood vessels. Several other characteristics of your baby's face and head give further evidence of your baby's tight squeeze through your birth canal: a flattened nose, ears pressed against the head, and a slight bruising of the skin over the prominent cheekbones. The watermelon shape of your baby's head is a result of a process called molding.

This elongated shape is necessary to help the head fit through your pelvic bones during delivery. As it enters the birth canal its bones move and allow the head to elongate to conform more easily to the shape of your birth canal. You may notice that your baby's skull bones overlap a bit so that they appear like ridges, especially on the top and sides of her head. Cesarean-delivered babies usually show less molding. You may feel your baby's "soft spot" (called a fontanel), a relatively soft area in the center top of your newborn's head where four of the skull bones join. This soft spot is actually covered by a thick membrane underneath, so it is okay to touch and wash this area. You may normally see and be able to feel a pulse through the soft spot. Occasionally tiny blood vessels break beneath the scalp during delivery allowing blood to accumulate and form a sort of goose egg on your baby's scalp. This is called a cephalohematoma. These normal bumps may take several months to disappear. Your newborn's scalp may be covered with fine silky hair, matted with amniotic fluid and specks of blood. You may also notice patches of fine furry hair called lanugo on the baby's earlobes, cheeks, shoulders, and upper back. Your newborn's soft skin is covered with a white, cheesy, slippery material called vernix, which protects it from the amniotic fluid and acts like a lubricant during vaginal delivery.

Your baby's eyes will be the most captivating part of your newborn's face. Within moments after birth newborns open their eyes in anticipation of meeting another pair of eyes. The puffy eyelids with the slit-like openings between them protect the sensitive newborn's eyes from too much light too soon. This is why it's a good idea to dim the lights after delivery, to encourage your baby to keep her eyes wide open and gaze at your faces. In the first few minutes after birth most newborns will open their eyes and gaze at their parents' faces for a few minutes. This is called the state of quiet alertness, which is a unique state in which babies are very receptive to their environment. Newborns seldom keep their eyes wide open for very long. Their heavy eyelids cause them to show intermittent periods of visual alertness, after which your baby will drift off into stages of deepening sleep.

Your baby should be dried with a towel immediately after birth to avoid evaporative heat loss, but don't be in a hurry to "clean" your baby. Enjoy your baby's unique newborn appearance immediately after birth, and after you have enjoyed a period of bonding (at least one hour) the attending personnel can then look after your baby and present to you a "picture book" baby.

13. *We are still undecided as to whether or not to have our baby circumcised. Can you give us some pros and cons to help us make the right decision?*

The American Academy of Pediatrics advises that routine circumcision is medically unnecessary and we agree with this decision. First the cons: Circumcision is a surgical procedure and generally a very safe one, but, as with any surgical procedure, there are occasional problems, such as injury to the shaft of the penis, bleeding, or infection. Circumcision without the use of an anesthetic clearly causes pain to the baby. Lastly, circumcised babies often experience more irritation to the tip of the penis from strong urine or abrasive diapers. Normally the foreskin covers the glans (the tip) of the penis and protects the glans from irritation.

Now the arguments in favor of circumcision: Parents feel the foreskin is easier to keep clean when the baby is circumcised. (Actually, this is not true—see question 15.) Parents want him to look like most of the other males in their circle or like dad. In response to this concern, I feel parents need not worry about the baby being different. If the current trend toward fewer circumcisions continues, our guess is that within the next decade about half the males will be circumcised and half will not. In our experience boys do not compare circumcised versus intact foreskins. Modern teenagers have a much more mature outlook about individual differences than we give them credit for.

Parents may worry about the possibility of the uncircumcised child needing circumcision later on when it is a much more painful procedure. It is true that some boys need circumcision when they are older, but it is rare. Even so, if circumcision is necessary later in childhood or adulthood, the boy is involved in the decision-making process and anesthesia is used. Except in cultural or religious customs, routine circumcision in newborns is unnecessary. Your decision for your baby should be given the same attention that you would give any other cosmetic surgery. (See question 14 anesthetic for circumcision.)

14. *We would like to have our baby circumcised, but don't want to put him through the pain. I've heard about using a local anesthetic. Is this possible?*

Yes. It is a myth that newborns do not feel pain during circumcision. Studies comparing the physiologic effects of circumcision on anesthetized and unanesthetized babies show the following: Babies who did not receive a local anesthetic cried more, developed higher heart rates, had higher levels of stress hormones, showed a drop in blood oxygen, and generally seemed much more stressed.

The procedure you refer to is called a dorsal penile nerve block, meaning that a small amount of xylocaine is injected just beneath the skin on both sides of the penis to numb the skin where the incision is made. I have personally used this technique on several hundred babies and have experienced no complications. (If your doctor is unaware of this technique, a description of the procedure is located in the following reference: *Journal of Pediatrics*, Vol. 92, p. 998.) While the number of circumcisions in the United States is gradually diminishing, many parents still prefer to have their baby circumcised although they do not want to inflict pain. A local anesthetic alleviates much of the pain for the baby—and the parents.

15. *We have chosen not to circumcise our child. How do we care for the foreskin?*

We call this the "uncare" of the foreskin. Unless your doctor, because of a medical problem, advises otherwise, simply leave the foreskin alone until it begins to retract naturally. If left alone, most foreskins naturally and very gradually retract until they are fully retractable around two to three years of age. Don't forcefully retract the foreskin. You may break the seal between the foreskin and the penis, allowing secretions to accumulate beneath the foreskin and result in infection. As the foreskin retracts naturally, wash out the secretions that may have accumulated beneath it. Teach your child to learn this hygiene as part of his bath-time routine. Sometimes tiny pockets of white secretions, called smegma, accumulate beneath the foreskin. If these secretions do not enlarge, are not infected, and do not seem to bother the baby, you can safely leave them alone. Sometimes applying warm compresses to the area dissolves the retained secretions. As the foreskin naturally retracts, you can then wash these secretions away. If your child later notices that he looks different than a circumcised friend, emphasize the positive aspects of his appearance by referring to his penis as "intact" rather than "uncircumcised."

16. *Could you explain what the routine injection and eye drops are that are given to baby after birth?*

After birth your newborn will be given an injection of Vitamin K because newborns may be deficient in this vitamin, which enables normal blood clotting. Your newborn will also be given some ointment in her eyes, usually erythromycin ointment, which will prevent an infection which might be caused by germs contacted during the passage through the birth canal. In order to enhance the bonding time with your baby immediately after birth, request that the attending medical personnel delay these routine procedures for several hours after delivery so as not to upset your baby or interfere with the eye-to-eye contact that you and your baby should enjoy right after birth.

17. *I've heard that right after birth our baby will be given a score that measures how healthy he is. What does that score mean?*

This score is called the *Apgar score*, developed by Dr. Virginia Apgar nearly thirty years ago. It is performed at one and five minutes after your baby's birth and is based upon five criteria: heart rate, breathing pattern, muscle tone, color, and general activity. Your baby gets from zero to two points for each of these. Please understand that the Apgar score was not meant to be given to parents and is not meant to be a valid score for the future health of the baby. A baby who scores a ten is not necessarily healthier than a baby who scores an eight. The Apgar score was designed to help the attending medical personnel know how to attend to the baby and decide how much observation he will need. A baby who scores lower than average may have temporary problems adjusting to life outside the womb and therefore is watched more carefully and given more assistance in the post-natal period of adjustment of her breathing and circulatory systems.

Studies have shown that except with very low scores, the Apgar score usually given to parents has no predictive validity toward the eventual health of the baby. For example, some babies cry a lot immediately after birth and therefore get two points for "a healthy cry." Some equally healthy babies assume a state of "quiet alertness" which is just as healthy and, in fact, more desirable than crying, although it does not rate points on the Apgar score. A low score should not be a source of anxiety, but simply alerts the attending personnel to observe the baby more carefully over the next few hours. Usually this observation does not have to result in separation from your baby, especially if you are in an LDR setting, where the nurse is assigned to care for and observe both mother and baby.

18. *Our hospital offers the options of taking care of our baby in the nursery or having our baby room in with us after delivery. I want rooming in. Which is better?*

Trust your feelings. Rooming in is definitely better. It means that you will be the primary care giver of your newborn, and the attending medical personnel assume the role of consultants and advisers to assist you. Nursery care means that your baby spends most of the time in the nursery and is brought in to you at scheduled times for feedings. In this case the nursery personnel are the primary care givers.

Rooming in is certainly the best for the following reasons: It allows you and your baby to develop an important quality of getting adjusted to each other which we call "harmony." You and your baby learn how to "read" each other. You learn to respond to your baby's cues. He then learns to cue better and you learn to respond better. Some mothers have been led to believe that they would get more rest if the baby is not in their room. On the contrary, in our experience mothers become anxious when separated from their babies. They feel they should be with him and often do not sleep as well when separated.

In our practice, we have studied the difference between the nursery-care situation and the rooming-in option and have found the following differences: When mothers and babies room in together, the mother's milk comes in an average of twenty-four to forty-eight hours sooner; the babies lose less weight; babies cry less; mothers leave the hospital much more confident in exercising their mothering skills; and the incidence of postpartum depression is lower. Studies have also indicated that the "fussy baby syndrome" occurs less often with babies who have roomed in with their mothers.

For the mother who is unable to room in with her baby because of a medical complication, we offer a word of reassurance. While rooming-in does enhance mother–infant bonding, this is not an instant glue which cements the relationship forever. Bonding is a lifelong process of being with and getting to know your baby. If you and your baby must be temporarily separated, delayed bonding can occur without any lasting effects on your relationship. The earlier and the more you are with your newborn, the faster you both get to know each other and the easier you get into mothering.

19. *What's going to happen with our newborn's umbilical cord, and how do I care for it?*

A baby's umbilical cord is usually cut and clamped about a half inch long. In the first few days your baby's cord may be swollen and jelly-like. It then begins to shrivel, dry, and will usually fall off within a week or two. The cord clamp is usually removed after twenty-four hours. To enhance the drying of the cord and prevent infection, clean the circumference around the base of the cord with a cotton-tipped applicator dipped in alcohol, or whatever antiseptic solution your doctor recommends. It is wise to continue cord hygiene even for a few days after the cord has completely detached. It is normal to see a few drops of blood the day the cord falls off. If the area around your baby's cord becomes red and swollen—about the size of a quarter—and/or your baby's cord develops an offensive odor, it may be infected and you should call your doctor.

20. *When our pediatrician takes care of our newborn in the hospital, what does she actually do?*

There are many behind-the-scenes activities that occur in the care of your newborn after birth. Much of this depends on your needs as a mother and your baby's general health. If your obstetrician expects or anticipates a problem at delivery, she may ask that your pediatrician attend the delivery to assist your baby in adjusting the heart and lung systems to a life of air breathing. After your baby is born and is deemed stable, meaning that the heart and lungs are working properly and breathing is normal, the pediatrician then does a head-to-toe examination to be sure all of your baby's organs are in the right place and are working properly. For example, the doctor examines your baby's hips to make sure that the thigh bones do not slip out of the hip sockets, a condition called dislocatable hips. This condition is easiest to detect during the immediate newborn period, but may be very difficult to detect later on when your baby's muscles tighten. Your doctor also checks to be sure the routine injections, eye medications, and blood tests have been performed and the results are normal. A nice custom which most mothers enjoy is requesting your doctor to examine your baby on your bed in your room. In watching the exam you will learn some interesting features about your newborn and appreciate more about what your doctor does. The doctor also checks the blood type of your baby to be sure that it is compatible with yours. If it is not, she is alerted to a potential problem that may or may not occur. Your baby's doctor can also assist you in feeding your baby. If you are bottle feeding, she will select the right formula for your baby. If you are breast-feeding, she will be sure you are instructed in proper positioning and latch-on techniques which are important to getting the breast-feeding relationship off to a smooth start. During your hospital stay, make a list of all the questions that you will want to ask your baby's doctor on the day of discharge from the hospital. When you sit down for your "going-home talk," be sure all your questions are answered and that you know how to reach your doctor should you have questions after going home.

21. *Our baby was just born two months prematurely. He had some breathing problems for the first few days but now seems to be doing well; however, the doctors say he will be in the hospital for at least a month to six weeks. I know he needs special care, but I feel left out as a mother. What can I do?*

Premature babies do need special care by a host of medical personnel, and they need it for a long time. It is easy for parents to feel left out of this inner circle that cares for the baby. However, you are a very important part of the medical team, if not the most important part. Here's how you can help care for your baby. First, realize that it is normal for you to psychologically distance yourself somewhat from your baby. Parents of premature babies often do this as a protective mechanism against the grief of possibly losing their baby. Since it seems that your baby is out of danger and will survive, it is now time to assume your rightful role as his mother. Rent an electric breast pump and pump your milk. Breast milk is especially valuable for premature babies both nutritionally and as protection against infections to which preemies are especially susceptible. Spend as much time as possible holding your baby. One of the recent advances in caring for premature babies is the finding that babies thrive (meaning growing to their fullest potential) better if they are frequently touched and rocked and sung to by their parents. Research has shown that babies who receive a lot of touching and rocking from their parents gain weight faster and leave the hospital sooner. Once your baby is off oxygen and intravenous support, try the custom of "packing." This recent innovation has also been shown to help preemies thrive. Packing means wrapping the infant securely around his mother's chest using a blanket or soft shawl. The baby is kept warm and has the benefit of skin-to-skin contact with your breasts. Walk around the nursery with your baby "packed" closely. Your warmth, your voice, your walking motion, which the baby has grown accustomed to for the past seven months, and your skin-to-skin touch all benefit your baby in a way that medical personnel cannot. As a matter of fact, you have the benefit of seeing your baby grow the final two months *outside* the womb. The more you participate in your baby's care, the more both of you will benefit. You should encourage dad to get involved in baby's care too. A hospital care-by-parent policy is not just a trend; it is good medicine.

22. *Could you explain the blood tests that are given to our baby before we leave the hospital?*

Just before leaving the hospital your baby will be given a blood test which screens for three possible illnesses. If detected early, all three are treatable, but if left undetected and untreated, they may cause harm to your baby. These three diseases are the following:

1. PKU (phenylketonuria), an extremely rare disorder occurring in approximately one in 15,000 infants. This disease is caused by the absence of a certain enzyme which is necessary to handle a normal protein called phenylalanine. If this protein builds up too high in your baby's blood it can cause brain damage. If PKU is detected early, however, it can be treated with a special diet.
2. Hypothyroidism. A drop of your baby's blood is also analyzed to be sure that she has sufficient thyroid hormones. If these are low, a general growth deficiency and possible brain damage can result. Congenital hypothyroidism occurs in approximately one out of 5,000 infants. This is actually the most important of the three tests.
3. Galactosemia. This disease is caused by a missing enzyme which is necessary for the proper metabolism of milk sugars. If the products of these sugars build up too high, they can damage many of your baby's vital organs. This disease is much more rare than the other two, occuring in approximately one in 60,000 infants. These screening tests are necessary and the results are automatically sent to your doctor within a week or two. Because these diseases are rare, do not be anxious that your baby might have one of them. All babies are screened in the hospital to pick up the one in thousands who might be vulnerable.

23. *Many of my friends' babies have developed jaundice a few days after birth. Is this normal? Can I do anything to prevent it from occurring in our expected baby?*

Most newborns develop a yellow coloring in the skin and eyeballs called jaundice. This condition is caused by the buildup in the blood of a yellow pigment called bilirubin, which is deposited in the skin. Newborns have excess red blood cells, and when these are broken down, they release substances which form bilirubin. Usually excess bilirubin is eliminated by the liver; however, many babies have a temporarily immature liver which is not able to handle this excess bilirubin. If too many red blood cells are broken down too fast or your baby's liver is unable to remove the excess bilirubin from the blood, jaundice appears.

There are two types of jaundice. For simplicity we will call them normal and abnormal jaundice. Abnormal jaundice may indicate that there is a difference in your baby's blood type and your blood type, causing too many blood cells to be broken down too fast, or that there is a problem in the infant's liver, or that there's some other problem with your baby's metabolism so that the excess bilirubin cannot be normally removed. Abnormal jaundice is quite rare. Normal jaundice is what most babies get because the liver is temporarily too immature to dispose of the excess bilirubin. Normal jaundice will not harm your baby. Your doctor will explain to you whether your baby has normal jaundice or abnormal jaundice, which may need treatment.

Occasionally, jaundice is caused by the baby not getting enough milk. The best way to prevent this type of jaundice is to room in with your baby and feed your baby on cue. Jaundice is often a needless source of anxiety for a new mother at a time when she is particularly vulnerable to any suggestion that her baby may not be completely normal. Be sure your doctor explains the cause of your baby's jaundice to you and sets your mind at rest about its transient nature. Jaundice in a healthy, full-term baby is rarely a cause for concern.

24. *We have a new baby and it seems I'm always changing diapers. What are his bowel movements supposed to look like, and how often should I expect them to occur?*

During the first few weeks a baby's stools change a lot. In the first few days they are black, tarry, and sticky, because they contain a lot of meconium which your baby had in his intestines while in the womb. Over the next few days the stools become greenish brown in color and less sticky. Between one and two weeks they take on a yellowish color and a pasty consistency. As the fat content of your milk increases, the stools of breastfeeding babies become yellow, seedy, and develop a mustard-like consistency and a not unpleasant aroma like buttermilk. Breast milk acts as a natural laxative so you can expect a breastfed baby's stools to be frequent and soft. Formula-fed babies have firmer, darker, and more odorous stools. If you are using an iron-fortified formula, expect your baby's stools to have a greenish color from the iron.

The number of stools a newborn baby has varies considerably. Some babies have a loose stool after every breast feeding, and you will sometimes hear the gurgly sound of a soft stool a few minutes into the feeding. If you hear an explosive sound and see a watery stool, it may mean your baby is sick or that something in your milk or the formula is irritating his intestine.

Formula-fed babies usually have fewer stools than breast-fed babies. You can also expect a change of stools with a change in diet. As you change from formula to cow's milk or add solid foods to your baby's diet, you can expect a change in the consistency, number, and color of your baby's stools. As your baby gets older and eats more solids, expect the stools to become firmer, darker, and less frequent.

25. *Our newborn has a hard time having a bowel movement. She strains a lot and sometimes we even notice a drop of blood on her diaper. How can we help her?*

Constipation is very uncomfortable for a newborn baby, and it sounds like your baby is truly constipated. Some formula-fed babies normally have a bowel movement only once a day or once every other day, but are not uncomfortable and often not constipated. Try the following: If you are formula-feeding, experiment with different formulas to see which one produces more frequent and softer stools. Watch for signs that your baby is about to have a bowel movement (drawing up of legs, facial grimaces, and signs of straining). When she begins to strain, insert a glycerine suppository (available without prescription at your drugstore) into your baby's rectum and hold it there for fifteen minutes by holding her buttocks together. This will soften the baby's stool and lubricate the rectal area to allow a smoother passage. The blood you noticed is probably due to a tiny tear, called a rectal fissure, in the lining of the rectum. This is very common with constipation. By keeping your baby's stools softer with dietary and stool-softening treatments, this fissure will heal. Formula-fed babies need to have extra water to help the intestines form a softer stool.

26. *We have a new baby and I'm trying to decide what type of medical care is best for him. Is it necessary for him to have checkups even though he seems well?*

Yes. The system of pediatric care that has been set up throughout North America works very well. During the first six months your doctor should check your baby every one or two months, depending on the health needs of your baby and your experience as a parent. These are called *well-baby* and later on *well-child* exams. These exams are important. During these checkups your doctor will answer any questions you have as a new parent, examine your baby, and detect any developmental problems that may occur and recommend any treatment that is necessary.

Preventative medicine is always the best. By detecting potential problems early, the treatment is much more successful and less costly in the long run. In addition, during these examinations your doctor will discuss nutrition, give immunizations, and offer any medical advice that helps to keep your child healthy. During these well-baby and well-child checkups your doctor also grows in his knowledge of you and your child. Seeing your child when he is well establishes an important reference point for a medical judgment if your child gets sick. Most pediatric practices follow the schedule recommended by the American Academy of Pediatrics: once a month for the first six months, then once at nine months, twelve months, fifteen months, eighteen months, two years, two and a half years, three years, and once a year thereafter.

27. *We are just about to bring our newborn home from the hospital. How much weight can I expect her to gain over the next few weeks?*

Newborns usually lose between five and eight percent of their birth weight (six to ten ounces) in the first week after birth. The reason for this is that babies are born with extra fluid and fat to tide them over until their mothers' milk can supply sufficient fluid and nutrition. There are many factors which affect the amount of weight a baby loses, or gains. Large babies who have a lot of extra fluid tend to lose more weight than small babies. We have noticed that babies born at home usually lose less weight than babies born in a hospital. This is probably not because of the location of the baby's birth, but rather because babies born at home are almost never separated from their mothers. Therefore, they tend to nurse more often and get more milk. Another factor influencing the amount of weight loss during the first week is how soon the mother's milk increases. Babies who room in with their mothers and breast-feed on cue lose less weight because the milk supply increases sooner. These babies also seem to get a higher-calorie milk. Babies who are often separated from their mothers during the first week or who are fed only according to a rigid schedule tend to lose more weight.

In addition to recording your baby's birth weight, you should record her weight upon her discharge from the hospital. This data will serve as an important reference point when your doctor checks your baby's weight one or two weeks later.

Following the initial normal weight loss, a newborn

should begin to gain weight around four to six days after birth. Breast-fed babies usually show a slower weight gain than formula-fed babies during the first two weeks. Thereafter, breast-fed babies and bottle-fed babies show similar weight gains, averaging around an ounce a day during the last two weeks of the first month. Most babies gain at least a pound to a pound and a half during the first month. Besides feeding and care practices, your baby's body type may influence her weight gain. Ectomorphs (recognized by their lean and lanky appearance, long fingers, and long, narrow feet), show a slower gain in weight and a proportionately greater increase in height than do babies who are mesomorph (medium build) or endomorph (short, pudgy hands and feet and shorter, wider fingers and toes).

28. *Our month-old baby has a rattling sound when he breathes. However, he seems happy and doesn't act sick. Is this a cold?*

Around the second month, babies often have a surge in saliva production, often making more than they can swallow. The excess saliva collects in the back of the throat, producing a gurgly sound. When you place your hand on your baby's chest or back, you may feel a rattle that you think is coming from within his chest. What you are feeling is air vibrating the pooled saliva in the back of your baby's throat. These sounds and vibrations are transmitted throughout the chest but are not coming from within the chest. This is not truly a cold and no medicine is necessary. Your baby will not choke on these secretions even though the noise he produces may be worrisome to you. With time he will learn to swallow this excess saliva, and these normal chest rattles will diminish. These saliva noises usually lessen when the baby falls asleep because babies produce less saliva when they sleep. As long as your baby looks and acts well, you should not be alarmed.

29. *Our two-week-old baby gets a stuffy nose often and seems very troubled by it. His nose is so tiny that it is difficult to clean out. Any tips?*

Whereas adults can breathe well through either nose or mouth, babies are called *obligate nose breathers*, meaning they are dependent on clear nasal passages to breathe effectively. Babies also have the tiniest nasal passages in those early months when they are most dependent on their nose to breathe, so it is important to keep your baby's nasal passages clear. Here's how to care for them. Eliminate environmental irritants such as linty bed clothing, feather pillows and comforters, dust collectors (fuzzy animals and toys), and pungent odors, such as perfumes and cigarette smoke, from your baby's environment. Your newborn's nose is particularly sensitive to environmental irritants. Keep the air in your bedroom humid, preferably around fifty percent humidity, especially in the winter months in homes with central heating, which tends to dry out and irritate the nasal passages. Here's a tip for keeping your bedroom both warm and comfortably humid. Turn off the central heat in your bedroom and use a warm mist vaporizer as a heat source. A simple, inexpensive warm mist vaporizer can heat an average-size bedroom from the heat released by the condensation of the warm mist, while at the same time providing a humid environment which your baby's nasal passages like (but your wallpaper might not!).

Since your baby cannot blow his nose, here's how to help him. Buy a brand of saline nose drops recommended for infants. Squirt a few drops into each nostril with a plastic dropper. These drops loosen the secretions and stimulate your baby to sneeze them out. Next, take a nasal aspirator (a rubber bulb syringe available at a drugstore) and *gently* suck out the loosened secretions. Expect your baby to protest during this procedure, but afterward to be much happier as she can now breathe more comfortably. Never use a cotton-tipped applicator to clean deep into the nose. A newborn's nasal passages are too small. A moistened cotton applicator may be safely used to wipe off dried secretions around the opening to the nostrils.

30. *Our newborn has a pimply-type rash all over his face. It looks terrible. What can we do?*

This is called *newborn acne*. Like teenage acne, it is probably caused by increased levels of hormones left over from prenatal life. Most babies also have tiny, whitish, pinhead-sized bumps called "milia," which are most prominent on the skin of the nose and are caused by plugged pores of the skin. These normal types of newborn facial rashes disappear with normal facial hygiene. Gently wash your baby's skin with warm water and a soft washcloth. Overly dry air, such as that caused by central heating, may tend to aggravate skin rashes in the infant. A baby's skin enjoys humidity. A humidifier in your baby's bedroom should help. Babies also get a prickly heat type of rash appearing on areas of the skin where there is excessive heat and retained moisture, such as behind the ears, in neck folds, and in areas of the trunk covered by excessively tight-fitting clothing. A mild baking soda solution (one teaspoon to a cup of water) will soothe and cool the skin, enabling this rash to disappear. You should also dress your baby in lighter-weight, looser-fitting clothing to avoid prickly heat (100 percent cotton is best).

31. *Our new baby's fingernails grow very fast, but I'm afraid to cut them. Could you give us some nail-cutting tips?*

Sometimes babies are born with fingernails so long that they need to be cut right away to prevent them from scratching their faces. It is easiest to trim a baby's fingernails while he is asleep. Use a small blunt-ended nail scissors specially designed for babies. A baby's toenails do not seem to grow as fast as the fingernails. You may notice that your baby's toenails seem to be ingrown into the sides of his toes, but this is not a cause for concern. Because a baby's toenails are so soft and flexible, ingrown toenails are seldom a problem.

32. *My baby's scalp has a lot of flaky stuff on it which is very hard to remove. How can I get rid of it?*

This condition is called *cradle cap*. Most babies have it. These crusty, oily plaques are very difficult to prevent and to remove if they are allowed to get too thick. First, gently massage vegetable oil, such as corn oil or olive oil, into the crusty areas. Next, gently remove the softened scales with a washcloth or soft bristle brush. In particularly thick areas you may wish to use a soft toothbrush. If the rash continues and develops into an especially thick crust, a prescription cream may be necessary. A tar-based shampoo can be effective in particularly severe cases; however, the greatest of care should be taken to avoid contact with the baby's eyes.

After you have removed all the cradle cap crust, take the following preventive measures: Increase the humidity in your baby's room to prevent dryness and flakiness of the scalp. Occasionally massage the oil into your baby's scalp and use a tar-based shampoo at the first sign of a recurrence of cradle cap. Some scalp rashes are particularly resistant and need consultation from your baby's doctor or a dermatologist. (See related question 34.)

33. *Our new baby's bones seem to crackle a lot when we move her, such as during diaper changes. Is this normal?*

Yes. The joints of tiny babies are composed of many tiny bones loosely held together by very stretchy ligaments. The crackles you hear are these tiny moving parts sliding on each other during limb movement. These joint noises are common, normal, and usually subside toward the end of the first year. Babies really are not fragile and you don't have to worry about these noises. Like most of the normal but worrisome noises of infancy, these too will disappear.

34. *How often should we bathe our newborn, and what type of soap should we use?*

Most babies are washed too much. Perhaps this reflects your mother-cat instinct. Bathing is really playtime; babies don't get dirty enough to need a daily bath. For busy parents, this is good news. Twice a week (especially in the winter) is enough bathing, provided you clean your baby's diaper area well every time there is a bowel movement.

If your baby's facial skin is extremely oily (baby acne), a little mild soap helps dry the excess oil and pimples. Use a mild soap, preferably one that contains moisturizing cream (such as Dove or Neutrogena). If your baby is prone to dry skin, called eczema, use soup very sparingly and blot skin dry. Too much soap and vigorous rubbing depletes the baby's skin of natural oils. Cotton-tipped applicators are handy in cleaning little crevices in and behind the outer ear, but never try to clean inside the ear canal, for you may cause damage to the canal or eardrum.

35. *My baby screams every time I try to give her a bath. What should I do?*

Since bath time should be fun time for both you and your baby, here are some tips on getting your baby clean and also enjoying this ritual: You need a warm, draft-free room, a basin of water, and a thick towel on which to place your baby. Many babies cry if you undress them completely, making bath time too upsetting for both of you. If this happens, undress and bathe the baby in stages. Other babies love the feeling of being free of clothing, and cry when you are ready to dress them. Immerse your baby slowly in warm water (pre-test the temperature of the water first with your hand). The warm water is a signal to the baby to relax her muscles and feel her buoyancy. You will see pleasure on her face, probably a smile, and little floating movements of her arms and legs. Give yourself and the baby lots of time to enjoy this ritual. There are several types of baby bathtubs on the market. Some you place on a tabletop or counter, others sit in your big bathtub, or you can simply use the kitchen sink, which makes great pictures for the baby book and really tickles the fancy of the older children. A little tip is to wear a pair of old white cotton gloves and rub a little mild baby soap on the wet glove. You have an instant washcloth that automatically shapes itself to the baby's body and reduces the slipperiness of bare hands on soapy skin. Also, place a towel on the bottom of the sink or tub to prevent him from slipping. When washing her face, just use water. Soap in the eyes can really hurt.

If your baby screams every time you try to put her into the water, it either means that she is hungry, the water is too hot or cold, or you have a baby who doesn't like to be alone in the water. Her security may be threatened. A beautiful solution is to take your baby into your bath with you. Get the water ready, a little cooler than you usually have it. Then undress yourself and undress your baby. Hold her close to you as you get into the water, and then sit back and enjoy this glorious skin-to-skin contact. If your baby still protests, sit in the tub first, showing that you are enjoying your bath. Then have someone else hand your baby to you while sitting in the bathtub. Don't be surprised if your baby wants to nurse at this time. It is a natural result of being close to your breasts. In fact, if your baby still fusses upon entering the water in your arms, put her to your breast first as you slowly ease your way into the bath. This is a special way to enjoy mothering and bathing your baby. As your baby gets older, bath toys such as the traditional rubber duckie may entice the reluctant bathtaker.

36. *I've heard that infant massage is good for babies. Can you give me some tips on massaging my baby?*

Yes, infant massage is good for your baby and fun for you. Babies love an oil massage. Undress your baby completely and sit on the floor with your baby lying on a thick towel on your outstretched legs. Use pure vegetable oil to lubricate your hands and gently massage baby's entire body. Massage from head to toe. Use a systematic, firm, gentle stroking. Very light touching irritates some babies. Conclude the massage ritual with some bending and stretching exercises. Both mother and father should massage baby as it is important for him to get used to the different touching of both parents. Many fathers in our practice use infant massage to relax their babies as an alternative to the relaxation of nursing. After a few weeks you may notice that your baby begins to relax as soon as you place him on the familiar towel and in the familiar massage position, as if he anticipates the pleasant ritual to follow. In recent years there has been much research confirming the therapeutic and relaxing value of touch. (See *Infant Massage* by Vimala Schneider McClure, Bantam Books, 1989.)

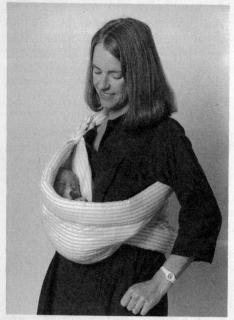

A sling-type carrier helps a mother remain close to her baby.

37. *I want to carry my baby close to me and am about to purchase a baby carrier. There are many different types on the market. Can you give me some advice on which one to choose?*

We call this parenting style "wearing your baby." It enhances development of the baby and makes life easier for mother and father. Consider the following in choosing a baby carrier: first of all, safety. Be sure the baby can be securely positioned in the carrier. Choose one that has been thoroughly tested by a reputable manufacturer. A great many baby carriers are being introduced, and we feel that some of them have not been adequately safety-tested. If you are being given a used carrier, be sure the straps and connectors are sturdy and properly attached. The leg openings should be large enough not to pinch, but small enough to keep the infant from falling out. Check for frayed straps, loose snaps, or ripped seams. Comfort, for both parents and baby, is an important consideration. Cotton, or cotton polyester blend, is the most comfortable and washable fabric. A well-designed carrier should evenly distribute your baby's weight on your shoulders and hips, not on your back and neck. It should be well padded over the shoulders and along the back and wherever the edges of the carrier press against the baby's torso and legs.

Choose a carrier that is versatile. To avoid having to purchase a series of carriers as your baby gets older, choose a carrier that can be used from birth to two years in various carrying positions. Choose a carrier that is easily adjusted while being worn so that your baby won't be unnecessarily disturbed. A fact of human nature is that if something is not convenient to use, we won't use it. Fathers especially shy away from carriers that have many sets of buckles and straps.

We have found the sling-type carrier (see photo) is the most versatile for accommodating a baby's changing size and development. In the early months, the infant can be cradled against his mother's chest (easier for discreet nursing) and later on can be carried on the hip, with his weight evenly distributed between the parent's shoulder and hip. Baby carriers are nurturing devices allowing you to "wear" your baby while still carrying on the busy life-styles that most parents have.

The brand we suggest is the Original Baby Sling by

Nojo Inc. (phone 1–800–854–8760 for your nearest store). See question 38 for more about wearing your baby.

38. *My friend not only carries her baby everywhere, but the baby is always in someone's arms. Isn't she going to spoil her baby? Will the baby ever learn to crawl?*

No, your friend is not spoiling her baby; and yes, he will learn to crawl and probably crawl better. New research is proving what experienced mothers have long known—that something good happens to parents and infant when the baby is carried a lot. Infant-development specialists, who travel throughout the world studying infant-care practices, have repeatedly observed that babies who are carried in a variety of cloth-type slings and carriers seem more content than infants who are kept in cribs, playpens, strollers, and prams. We feel it is much better for a baby to be worn than wheeled. Baby wearing is not a fad of the 90s; we think it is likely to continue to be popular for two reasons: Parents want to do whatever they can to enhance their baby's development, but they also have busy life-styles. Wearing your baby accommodates both needs. Mothers in other cultures have fabricated various carriers out of necessity because they're constantly on the go. Mothers in Western cultures are also on the go a lot—they must "go" differently. For example, I, Martha, am a lactation consultant and teach breastfeeding classes. One day before one of my seminars, our then six-month-old, Matthew, developed an ill-timed fussy period. Not wishing to cancel my class, but also not wanting to leave Matthew with a baby-sitter during a high-need period, I "wore" him in a sling while delivering a one-hour lecture to one hundred and fifty pediatricians. After I finished my talk on parenting styles, a doctor came up to me and exclaimed, "What you did made more of an impression than what you said!"

Two years ago we attended an international parenting conference. Noticing that many mothers from Third World countries wore their babies in sling-type carriers which looked like an extension of their own clothing, we asked these mothers why baby wearing was so popular in their culture. We received very simple answers: "It makes life easier for the mother." "It's good for the baby." Over decades of tradition other cultures have learned that carried babies thrive better. All babies grow, but not all babies thrive. Thriving means growing to one's fullest potential, not only getting taller and wider but growing in behavioral competence. We don't believe that there is any mysterious scientific reason why carried babies thrive better. If a baby wastes less energy crying, he has more energy left over to grow and develop—to thrive.

Several years ago during research and preparation for our book *The Fussy Baby*, I noticed that the more babies were carried, the less they cried. Mothers of fussy babies would commonly say, "As long as I wear him, he's content!" Based on these observations we began advising parents in our practice to carry their babies as much as possible right after coming home from the hospital. I advised them to get a sling-type carrier and adjust the sling and the baby to a position that was most comfortable for both of them. This is why we call it baby wearing—you adjust the baby and the carrier to the proper fit, much as you would a piece of clothing. We kept careful notes over a period of three years. Our studies show that carried infants cried much less, showed fewer colicky episodes, and seemed more content. Carrying creates an environment which lessens the baby's need to cry.

Carrying probably settles babies partly by its effect on their vestibular system. This system, located behind each ear, is similar to three tiny carpenter's levels, one oriented for side-to-side balance, another for up-and-down, and the third for back-and-forth. When baby is carried, he moves in all three of these directions. They all function together to keep the body in balance. Every time you move, the fluid in these "levels" moves against tiny hair-like filaments which vibrate and send nerve impulses to the muscles in your body that keep you in balance. The pre-born baby has a very sensitive vestibular system which is constantly stimulated because the fetus is in almost continuous motion. Carrying "reminds" the baby of the womb. Motion is the normal way of life for babies, not stillness.

Carried babies also have a head start on learning. A baby who's carried more cries less and spends more time in a state of quiet alertness (also called interactive quiet). This is the behavior state in which a baby is most receptive to and interactive with his environment. This is why some researchers report enhanced visual-auditory alertness in carried babies.

Carrying humanizes a baby. Carried babies become more aware of the parent's face, of her walking rhythm, voice, and scent. Carried babies are intimately involved in their parents' world because they participate in what their mother or father is doing. A baby "worn" while his mom washes dishes, for example, hears, smells, sees, and experiences in depth the adult world. Very simply, the baby is more exposed to and involved in what's going on around him.

Of course, parents have to put their babies down sometimes! In fact, it is important to take a balanced approach to baby wearing. This style of parenting means changing our mindset regarding what babies are really like. New parents may think of the picture-book baby as one who lies quietly in a crib, gazing passively at dangling mobiles, only picked up to be fed, played with, and then put down. They may think that "up" periods are just dutiful intervals to quiet the baby long enough to put him down again. The concept of baby wearing reverses this view: Babies are carried much of the time, and put down long enough for nap times, sleep, and for parents to attend to their own needs. "Down babies" learn to cry to get picked up. "Up babies" learn non-crying body language to signal their need to get down. The amount of carrying naturally decreases as the baby increases in age and motor skills. However, even a toddler may show occasional high-need periods when he wants to be picked up and held close.

Some babies need more carrying than others. Certain babies, whom we call high-need babies (a nicer term than fussy babies, although it means the same thing) settle quite nicely when carried. These babies have a tendency to stiffen, arch, and seem to be doing back dives. They profit from the bending position that carrying gives, and they enjoy the closeness of being wrapped around their mother's or father's body. Like so many parenting styles, no single method works all the time. Parents may more easily survive their high-need baby if they consider "gestation" of a baby as eighteen months—nine months inside the womb and nine months more outside the womb but not far away from the security and comfort of a parent.

Mothers do not have a patent on baby wearing. As the father of seven and a certified baby wearer, I, William, feel that a baby gets used to a father's handling too. Babies enjoy this different type of stimulation. It is not better or less than mom's, it is different. And often the vibration of a deeper male voice while father talks and sings to the baby will lull a fussy infant back to sleep.

Baby carriers are nurturing devices which make rediscovering the lost art of wearing the baby easier for parents—and a good time to be a baby.

39. *I'm having difficulty getting close to our month-old baby. I've heard so much about babies just melting and molding into a parent's arms and loving to be picked up. My baby doesn't like to be held; she acts as if when she's older, she will say to me, "Mom, as soon as I'm old enough to feed and dress myself, you're fired." How can I get closer to her?*

Your baby is one of the special babies whom we call non-cuddly babies. The textbook baby loves to cuddle and loves to be picked up and held. Some babies come wired with a certain temperament that makes them slow to warm up to their care givers. This can be very frustrating to a new mother. Above all, this is not your fault. Your style of mothering does not make your baby this way; it is only your baby's unique temperament. Your baby will eventually want to be held and cuddled, but perhaps not as much as other babies do.

Try the following: Slow-to-warm-up babies often prefer to be carried in the bent position, either backward facing with their legs up against your chest and your arms embracing their back and looking them straight in the eye or forward facing with back and head resting against your chest and your arms cradling their thighs so they face outward. These babies often arch their back and push out of your arms when being held too tightly. This is why holding them in the facing-outward position is usually better. With time, the tonic-muscle reflexes that tend to cause a baby to hold her muscles tight and to arch her back tend to relax (usually around three to four months), at which time she may be less stiff, easier to bend, and snuggle in to the contours of your body, and she may actually like to be held. Try a sling-type carrier which allows the baby to be cradled across your chest or to face outward to see the world. The carriers which make her lie flat against your chest are often too confining for these types of babies. A gentle oil massage often helps warm up the baby to like to be touched. (See question 36 for infant massage techniques.) A warm bath together will often help soothe a difficult-to-cuddle baby. Remember go gently and gradually in loosening up this type of baby. (See questions 37, 38 for tips on selecting a carrier for this type of baby.)

40. *Our three-week-old baby's eyes often seem to be tearing, and we have noticed yellow matter accumulating. What should we do?*

It sounds as if your baby has blocked tear ducts. Around three weeks of age most infants begin tearing. Normally these tears drain through a tiny canal between the nasal corner of your baby's eye and the nose. If these tear ducts are blocked, tears will back up into his eyes and become infected. This is not a serious problem, and you can do the following to help. Wash the yellow matter out with clear water. Gently massage with your fingertip (provided it is clean and that one fingernail has been cut very short) at the nasal corner of the eye where the lower eyelid meets the bridge of the nose. Massage *toward* the nose. Do this a half-dozen times before each diaper change. If the discharge is becoming thicker and yellower, consult your doctor about a prescription eye ointment to treat the infected tears. Blocked tear ducts, if properly treated, usually open up by six months. If not, an eye doctor may need to open up the tear ducts by probing into the ducts with a tiny wire. This procedure is not serious and can often be done in the doctor's office.

41. *Is it better to put our newborn down to sleep on her stomach or her back?*

Newborns usually sleep better on their stomachs than on their backs. Some mothers feel that the reason for this is that a newborn feels more helpless when awaking on her back, perhaps the way a turtle feels when turned over. When on her stomach, even a newborn has the strength to lift her head and turn herself a bit with her arms. Newborns also breathe more efficiently while lying on their stomachs.

When falling asleep shortly after a feeding, a baby is best placed on her side to sleep. Roll up a towel and wedge the towel in the crevice between the baby's back and the mattress. Position your baby on her right side, for this allows the stomach to empty by gravity.

After the first few weeks babies seldom remain long on their sides but roll onto their stomachs to sleep. When placing your baby down to sleep, turn her head to one side. Don't worry about her suffocating. Even a newborn is able to lift her head just far enough to turn it to one side or another. Instead of placing your baby in the center of the crib, place her touching one side. Babies like the security of sleeping against some object or person. This explains why they often squirm their way into the corner of the crib as if trying to find a corner of their new womb in which to snuggle. When your baby is sleeping on her stomach, pull her legs out from under her and turn them outward. Babies tend to sleep in the fetal position with their legs tucked upward and inward under their abdomen. This position tends to prolong the normal bowlegged tendencies of babies.

42. *We have a one-month-old baby. How should I dress him at night, and how warm should we keep his room?*

Most babies are overdressed. Dress and cover your baby in as much or as little clothing as you would yourself plus one more layer. If your baby was premature, weighs under ten pounds, or has little insulating body fat, dress him even more warmly. Cotton clothing is best because it absorbs body moisture and allows air to circulate freely. Your baby's clothing should be loose enough to allow free movement, but well-fitting enough to stay on the proper body parts. Sleepers that contain foot coverings as part of the sleeper are usually best but may be more difficult to maintain a proper fit. If your baby's sleepers do not contain feet, clothe these cold little feet with white cotton socks. Avoid dangling strings or ties on your baby's sleepwear (and yours as well), since this could cause strangling.

Concerning the temperature of your baby's room, the consistency of the temperature is more important than how hot or cold it is. Premature or small babies have incompletely developed temperature-regulating systems and need reasonably consistent temperatures. Full-term healthy babies and older infants are better able to tolerate some degree of temperature swings. In the first few weeks babies do not easily adjust to marked swings in room temperature, so a consistent temperature around 70° F. (21° C.) is preferable. Attempt a relative humidity around fifty percent, which is best maintained by a warm-mist vaporizer during the winter months. Babies enjoy a relatively humid sleeping environment. A higher humidity tends to stabilize the room temperature in addition to maintaining the room heat. If you do use a vaporizer, clean it weekly to remove allergens such as mold. If your bedroom is cool, put a well-fitting nightcap on your baby's head during those early months when most babies do not have much insulating hair.

43. *Our two-year-old stands up in her crib and tries to climb out. How do I know when her crib is no longer safe and I should get her a bed?*

Place your baby's crib mattress in the lowest position. If her chin is above the level of the rail when she is standing erect and flat-footed, your baby is too tall to be safely left alone in the crib. Here are some other crib safety tips: To prevent scratching your baby and catching her clothing, metal hardware should be smooth and should not protrude into the crib. The baby should not be able to release the latches from the inside. Avoid placing large blocks and toys in the crib that could serve as steps for your infant to climb out of it. Do not place the crib against a window, near any dangling ropes, such as venetian blinds, or near any furniture which could be used to help the infant climb out. Avoid cribs with ornate tops. Infants have strangled in the concave space between the post and the crib. Cribs manufactured within the past ten years are highly regulated by the U.S. Safety Commission. Pamphlets concerning crib safety are available from the U.S. Consumer Products Safety Commission, Washington, D.C. 20207, or call toll-free 800–638–2666.

44. *Our baby has a bad diaper rash. What should I do?*

Diaper rashes are a normal occurrence when you put sensitive skin and diapers together. Diaper rashes are caused by the chemical irritation of urine and the mechanical rubbing of diapers. When urine stays in the diaper for a time, bacteria react with the urine to form ammonia, which acts as a chemical irritant to the skin and accounts for the pungent odor.

Here are some tips on lessening the frequency of your baby's diaper rash: Change him as often and as quickly as possible. Try to detect if the diaper is wet or dirty by how he acts or by the odor produced. After changing the diaper, rinse his diaper area with water with or without a mild soap and blot dry with a soft cloth. Don't use a strong soap or excessively rub the already sensitive skin. You may even allow your baby's diaper area to dry awhile before putting on another diaper. Exposing his diaper area to air and a bit of sunshine is a good diaper rash preventative. When your baby is asleep, let him lie bare bottom up and place a diaper underneath to catch urine. Avoid tight-fitting, elasticized diapers and rubber pants, which retain mositure and prevent the skin from breathing. Instead, use waterproof mats to protect bedding.

Experiment with both cloth and disposable diapers to see which one is most comfortable and least rash-producing for your baby. If you use disposable diapers, be sure to fold the edges of the diaper down so that the polyethylene lining does not touch and irritate the skin around the belt line.

Diaper rash should be treated early before the skin barrier is broken down and becomes infected. Once you notice the first signs of irritation (reddening of the skin), apply a barrier cream such as zinc oxide. Expect your baby to be more prone to diaper rashes during colds, teething, diarrhea, and antibiotic treatment. Use a barrier cream in these situations. If his diaper rash is raised off the skin, pustular, rough, or getting worse, consult your doctor for a prescription medication.

2

BREASTFEEDING

Questions about breastfeeding ranked second only to questions about sleeping problems in our listing of the types of questions that we received. This is because in the past ten years, more and more mothers have started breastfeeding their babies. They are finding they are doing so, however, in a culture which does not always support breastfeeding and is not well informed on how to help the new breastfeeding mother. In my experience as director of the Breastfeeding Center in San Clemente, California, I have found that most mothers intellectually want to breastfeed but emotionally are not prepared for the time and commitment this style of feeding requires during the early weeks. Fortunately, many support groups are now available to help the nursing pair get the right start. The largest, most experienced of these groups is the La Leche League, International. This is a volunteer organization composed of women members and group leaders, all of whom strongly advocate the league's motto: "Good mothering through breastfeeding." Each leader, in addition to having practical breastfeeding experience, has special training in counseling new mothers on breastfeeding and common concerns of child care. League mothers enjoy access to a lending library, a board of medical consultants, and continual input from other members through monthly meetings. There are approximately 13,000 league leaders and 4,200 league groups in 45 countries. (See Appendix, page 280 for information on how to locate your nearest LLL group.)

The most recent help for breastfeeding mothers is a new specialist called a lactation consultant. This is a woman who takes certified courses in teaching breastfeeding techniques and solving breastfeeding problems and who is certified by a board of examiners. The largest organization of lactation consultants is the International Board of Certified Lactation Consultants. Usually local hospitals will have a list of certified lactation consultants in your area.

Our main goal in this chapter is not only to encourage a mother to breastfeed, but to help her enjoy this relationship. You will spend more time feeding your baby than any other interaction during the first year or two—we want you to enjoy it.

45. *I think I want to breastfeed because it seems like most mothers are doing it now, but I'm not sure. Does it really make a difference?*

Yes! In addition to being good for the mother, the advantages of breastfeeding for a baby are even more impressive. Your milk, like your blood, is a living substance. Long ago, mother's milk was known as "white blood." Your milk is custom-made, beginning with colostrum—the special substance present in your breasts during pregnancy and in the first few days after birth before it changes to milk. Colostrum, your baby's first immunization, provides heavy doses of immunity from disease. It is a protein-rich food similar to the nourishment received through your placenta and a natural laxative to clear the meconium from baby's intestines. Each species supplies milk that is specific to the needs of its young. For example, the milk of cows is high in minerals and protein because rapid bone and muscle growth is necessary for a calf's mobility and survival. Human milk contains special proteins designed to promote brain growth, the survival organ of our species. All of the necessary elements are there in just the right proportion—fats, sugars, proteins, minerals, iron, vitamins, and enzymes. The special sucking action required during breastfeeding enhances the development of baby's oral muscles and facial bones.

The physical advantages to the baby are impressive enough, but when we look at the emotional advantages to a mother and baby, the case for breastfeeding is even more encouraging. Studies have shown that skin-to-skin contact and touching benefits a baby's physical, mental, and emotional development. Fresh from the tension of birth, a baby put to his mother's breasts hears her familiar heartbeat, her familiar breathing, her familiar voice; he feels the enveloping warmth and touch of her body; his mouth has a place to suck which helps the tension subside. His mother's face is right there, just at the right distance, hovering eight to twelve inches from a baby's face so that his eyes can drink in who she is even as he drinks in the colostrum. He is secure, he is home, and all is well.

Before you make your final decision, attend a couple of La Leche League meetings to find out the advantages of breastfeeding for a mother, baby and family. An important point to consider is what breastfeeding does for *you*. Many mothers consider breastfeeding as all giving, giving, giving. To a certain extent this is true early on—parents are givers and babies are takers. This is a realistic and exhausting fact of early parenting.

However, when you breastfeed your baby, he gives something back to you. When he sucks from your nipples, he stimulates a hormone called prolactin to enter your bloodstream. Prolactin, called the mothering hormone, helps a mother feel more nurturing. In fact, when prolactin was experimentally injected into male animals, they acted like mothers. This hormone also relaxes women. Busy mothers in our practice have confided that when they feel tense they simply nurse their babies, so many people feel that this hormone is the biological basis of the term *mother's intuition.* Breastfeeding is a mutual giving whereby your baby actually helps you to mother him. I also think of prolactin as a perseverance hormone which helps you get through those trying days. If you are still undecided at the birth of your baby, I advise you to commit yourself to a thirty day trial period of breastfeeding.

46. *We are expecting our first baby in a few months and really want to breastfeed. However, some of my friends have had so many problems breastfeeding that I am a little afraid I may not be able to. Could you give me some tips on getting off to the right start?*

I am glad that you used "we" in discussing your wish to breastfeed, because a father has a major role in insuring the success of breastfeeding. Breastfeeding is a life-style, not just a method of feeding. When you realize how breastfeeding benefits a mother, baby, and family, you will be more determined to overcome any difficulties that may arise in the early days or weeks of your breastfeeding experience.

In looking over the patients in our breastfeeding clinic, we have noticed that mothers who have successfully breastfed their babies have taken the following steps that we call our prescription for successful breastfeeding:

1. Prenatal breastfeeding education: During your pregnancy, surround yourself with experienced breastfeeding mothers by joining your local La Leche League, and purchase some of their books and pamphlets. Take a breastfeeding class.
2. Room in with your baby during your hospital stay.
3. Don't schedule: Watch your baby's cues, not the clock.
4. Seek help from a lactation consultant within the first forty-eight hours. This helps you and your baby develop

proper positioning and latch-on techniques before poor sucking habits and breastfeeding problems occur.

5. Surround yourself with a supportive environment of breast-feeding mothers and avoid negative advisers.
6. Father involvement: Get your husband to practice care and feeding of the breastfeeding mother.
7. Share sleep with your baby.
8. Avoid supplemental formula unless prescribed by your baby's doctor for a medical reason.

If you follow these eight steps during the early weeks, you are more than likely to enjoy and be successful at breastfeeding.

47. *I am expecting a baby in a few months and plan to breastfeed. Should I be preparing my nipples now, during my pregnancy, to prevent soreness?*

Lactation specialists feel that for most women, nipple-preparation exercises are not necessary. Women with fair skin, especially redheads, may experience more difficulty with nipple soreness. Some mothers have found that it helps to devote some time to conditioning their nipples during the last months of pregnancy by allowing gentle friction on the nipples at regular intervals over a long period of time to toughen them. Do this by wearing a nursing bra and dropping the flaps to expose your nipples to the gentle friction of your clothing. Frequent exposure of your nipples to air and briefly to sunshine is also a good way to condition your nipples. Do not remove the natural oils in your areola with soap. Plain water is sufficient. And read the next question.

48. *I am expecting a baby in three months, and my nipples seem to be somewhat flat. Will they gradually come out more, or should I be doing something now to help them protrude?*

Even nipples that look perfectly normal can flatten when tested. Ask your doctor or Lactation specialist to examine your breasts to determine whether your nipples are inverted (when the breast is compressed one inch back from the nipple, the nipple itself either flattens or goes in rather than shaping outward). Normally there is a lot of elastic and erectile tissue in your areola and nipple, which allows your baby to stretch the nipple into the back of her mouth during sucking. Some women have a different type of elastic tissue in their nipples. This causes the nipples to invert, or turn in, when stimulated rather than to become erect. Inverted nipples are difficult for baby to grasp.

If your nipples are inverted, the lactation specialist may recommend nipple stretching exercises and/or advise you to wear a breast cup throughout the rest of your pregnancy in order to help your nipples protrude. You may also need extra help getting your baby to latch on at first.

49. *I am two months pregnant and our two-year-old is still nursing occasionally. Is this all right? Can you give me some medical advice on whether or not it is safe to continue nursing our toddler during my pregnancy?*

Most obstetricians caution mothers about breastfeeding during pregnancy. In theory, breastfeeding stimulates a hormone (oxytocin) to be secreted into your bloodstream that would create contractions in your uterus. Now, however, obstetricians know that the oxytocin receptors in the uterus are not activated until the twenty-fourth week. At that point, *if* you are at risk for pre-term labor, there must be no nipple stimulation whatsoever. Many mothers successfully breastfeed throughout their pregnancy without any harm to either mother or baby. If you have a history of previous late miscarriages (after twenty weeks) or are experiencing contractions of your uterus during breastfeeding, it is wise to stop. The wisest course is to check with your doctor about whether it is safe to breastfeed in your particular case.

Many mothers experience heightened nipple tenderness during pregnancy, making breastfeeding uncomfortable. Limit the time your toddler spends actually sucking if you need to. Also, you can expect your milk to change taste during the final three months. Nursing toddlers commonly give "don't like anymore" signals during this time and wean themselves.

50. *Our six-week-old baby wants to nurse all the time, day and night. Frankly, I am exhausted and I'm not getting anything done. How can I get a break?*

In the first few months babies have "frequency days" when all they want to do is nurse. This is called marathon nursing. The supply-and-demand principle of breastfeeding is working in response to the fact that your baby is going through a growth spurt. He nurses more in order to stimulate your body to produce more, so he can grow more. Your baby may also be going through a period of high need. Some babies, whom we call high-need babies, want to be held "all the time" and nursed "all the time" during the first few months as they slowly become adjusted to life outside the womb.

Here are some survival tips: During high-need days, temporarily shelve all of your outside commitments which may drain your energy. Your baby is a baby for a very short time, and no one's life is going to be affected if the housework doesn't get done on time. In our experience, mothers become burned out not so much because of the demands of their baby, but because of too many other family commitments. Be sure your baby is getting mostly milk at each feeding and not a lot of air. Be sure your baby is latching on to your areola and has a good seal. Burp him well during and after a feeding. Use the burp and switch technique to attempt to get more of the higher-fat milk into your baby to satisfy him longer. Get used to "wearing" your baby in a sling or front carrier. This not only makes nursing more accessible, but it may satisfy your high-need baby if he wants the comfort of your closeness more than extra nursing. Avoid the filler-food fallacy. You may be advised to give your baby a supplemental bottle or cereal with the

implication that you don't have enough milk. This is usually
not necessary. Your baby is simply signalling that he needs
to nurse more, and you need to increase your level of supply
to meet his level of need. Sleep when your baby sleeps and
don't be tempted to "finally get something done." You need
to recharge your own system to cope with these high-need
periods. If things don't get better in a few days, consult a
lactation consultant.

51. *We are adopting a newborn. I have heard that it is
possible to breastfeed an adopted baby. Is this true?*

Yes, you can breastfeed your adopted newborn even if you
have never been pregnant yourself. However, you should
bear in mind that it requires much preparation, experience,
and expert consultation. Sometime within the month before
you expect to receive your baby, seek consultation from a
lactation specialist or a breastfeeding clinic that has had
experience in helping adoptive mothers breastfeed. To prepare your breasts, rent a good electric breast pump. Pump
your breasts about every three hours during the day. Next,
begin feeding your newborn right after delivery. If necessary check into the hospital yourself. Even better, if the
infant is medically well, take her home from the hospital as
soon as possible. You must begin feeding at your breast
before the baby has a chance to get hooked on a bottle and
develop nipple confusion. You probably won't have milk for
several weeks, so your baby will need a supplemental formula, and this is where the interesting part of breastfeeding
an adopted baby occurs. Your lactation specialist will fit you
with a supplemental nutrition system composed of a small
plastic container that fits onto your bra into which formula
is poured. A tiny tube comes from the container and rests
over your nipple. When the baby sucks from your breasts
she gets the formula through the tube. Be prepared to
temporarily dislike all the gadgetry that you must initially
use. While you will never fall in love with these machines,
you will gradually notice these gadgets less and your breast-

feeding baby more. The important fact is that she is sucking from your breast. This continued sucking gradually brings your milk in and decreases the amount of supplemental formula needed. Don't worry about how much milk you will eventually produce because some mothers, at best, produce only about half of their baby's nutritional needs. The closeness of the breastfeeding experience and the fact that your baby is stimulating your maternal hormones by sucking are the main benefits of breastfeeding an adopted baby.

52. *Our baby is three weeks old and all he does is nurse day and night. I feel tied down and physically drained. I love our tiny son, but quite honestly, I'm not enjoying motherhood as much as I thought I would. I am a thirty-year-old ex-career woman, and this is our first child. I guess that intellectually I was prepared for breastfeeding and stay-at-home motherhood, but emotionally I wasn't. Can you help me?*

Your feelings are shared by countless other mothers who approach motherhood with the same professional commitment as they did their previous career. You immerse yourself in mothering only to find yourself in over your head. Here are some adjustment tips:

The first month is a dramatic adjustment period for mothers and babies. In your previous career you were used to being in control, and you were able to predict and structure your time. You had organized daytime and nighttime schedules and probably experienced the "we can have it all" feelings of many childless couples. Suddenly a baby arrives to turn your life upside down. The first month is really a period for you and your baby to get used to each other. You are just beginning to develop realistic expectations based on how babies really are: They do get their days and nights mixed up; they do feed frequently and erratically; they do want and need to be held most of the time; and they frequently protest vehemently when separated from you. In essence, you went from an organized life-style to a disorganized one at the same time that your body went through tremendous adjustment changes. You may also be blessed with a baby with high needs, who takes a bit longer than usual to adjust to life outside the womb. We would like you to feel tied together to your baby, not tied down. Wear your baby in a comfortable infant carrier and take walks in the park. You don't have to stay in the house all the time with a new baby (unless medically advised). Home to a tiny baby is where you are, and babies are very portable in the early months. Surround yourself with experienced mothers who seem to enjoy mothering and allow yourself to profit from their advice. Ventilate your feelings and frustrations to trusted friends, especially your husband. Have realistic expectations of how much you can handle and don't be afraid to ask for help. The first month is the toughest. Your baby will gradually become more organized and less demanding. It does get easier.

53. *During the winter months I often get colds for which my doctor prescribes medicines. This winter I'm breastfeeding. I don't want to do any harm to my baby. Which medicines can I safely take?*

Most medicines are perfectly safe while you are breastfeeding, especially over-the-counter medications. In addition, antibiotics are safe to take during breastfeeding. Decongestants are safe if taken a couple of times a day for no more than two or three days in a row. With some decongestants you may notice your baby becoming hyper irritable, colicky, and sometimes sleepier than normal, or you may notice your milk diminishing somewhat. It's okay to use these cold remedies judiciously. Pain relievers such as aspirin and acetaminophen, if taken in moderation, are also safe. You're right to raise the question, however; it is important to check with your doctor before taking medicines while breastfeeding.

54. *My little girl is eight months old this week. She's teething and now she has discovered biting my breast! I've tried putting my fingers on her two bottom teeth and going, "No, No," or I will just tap her little mouth and go, "No, No," but she merely starts giggling. What can I do?*

I, Martha, have survived fourteen years of nursing our seven little biters. The usual reaction is to pull the baby away from the breast and scream, "No!" Some babies go on a nursing strike because some mothers are so violent in their reaction to being bitten, for which you can hardly blame the mother, especially if it's a hard bite. Some of the tykes really go at it and draw blood. Instead, try this: Pull your baby in really close to you when you sense her teeth coming down to bite. Draw her right in to your breast. She will automatically let go in order to open her mouth more or to uncover her nose. You don't have to disengage yourself from the clenched teeth. Your baby should lessen her bite as she realizes that something is different in her latch-on and she needs to adjust it. It's also okay to say no because they can understand that some undesirable reaction occurs when they bite. Try your best not to screech in agony because you can startle your baby enough to put her off nursing for a few days. I've had that happen to mothers I've worked with. Keep a record of when she usually bites. If she is doing it at the end of the feeding, interrupt the feeding before she has a chance to bite. Also, keep some teething toys in your freezer, such as a wet washcloth or a frozen banana and let her chomp on these toward the end of the feeding, or before the feeding if she chomps then. These techniques, plus saying, "Ouch, that hurts Mama!" will help preserve your breasts and teach your baby at the same time.

55. *I've heard that breastfeeding can be used as a natural contraceptive. How reliable is this method?*

Studies have shown that this natural method of birth control is around ninety-five percent effective *as long as certain rules are followed*. These rules are as follows:

1. Unrestricted breastfeeding without regard to daytime or nighttime scheduling.
2. Sleep with your baby and allow unrestricted night nursing.
3. Don't use a pacifier or water bottle. Sucking at the breast is better for the baby and is part of the natural spacing effect.
4. Delay artificial feedings until at least six months. Solid foods should not substitute for breastfeeding but rather add to the baby's overall food intake.
5. Don't overuse baby-sitters. Keep it under two hours. Better yet, just take the baby with you.

Studies have shown that almost all mothers who practiced these feeding styles are infertile for an average of thirteen to sixteen months. The reason that this method often does not work in our Western society is that we are oriented toward day feeding, night sleeping, and scheduled meals. Parents often don't follow these rules. It is interesting to see how the contraceptive effect of breastfeeding works. When your baby sucks at your breast, he stimulates the production of the mothering hormone, prolactin. The high level of prolactin circulating in your blood suppresses the levels of estrogen and progesterone, the hormones necessary for ovulation and the preparation of the womb for implantation of a fertilized egg. When ovulation does not occur and there are no changes in the lining of your uterus, you do not have menstrual periods and are infertile. As breastfeeding lessens and weaning approaches, the baby sucks less often and your level of prolactin falls. Your estrogen and progesterone levels rise. Your first postpartum menstrual period occurs, signaling that you are or soon will be fertile again. Shortly after this "warning menses," ovulation resumes and fertility returns. The amount of sucking stimulation and the level of prolactin required to suppress these reproductive hormones vary from woman to woman. In general, you are not fertile until after your first menstrual period occurs. A small percentage of women (around five percent) become fertile while breastfeeding according to the rules, before the warning menses occurs. If you wish to space your children it is not wise to rely only on breastfeeding as a contraceptive once your baby begins lessening the frequency of feedings, sleeping through the night, or starts solid foods. (For more information on natural family planning, contact the Couple to Couple League in your area. See Appendix, page 281.)

56. *I am three months pregnant and still nursing our high-need two-year-old. She shows no signs of wanting to wean and I really am not anxious to wean her. My heart tells me she is simply not ready yet, and my doctor has given me the go-ahead to continue breastfeeding. What can I expect?*

We certainly support your intuitive feeling that your two-year-old is not ready to wean. In fact, the best way to lessen sibling rivalry is not to wean the older child before her time. In reality, there are three needs to consider here: those of your pre-born baby, those of your health, and the emotional needs of your two-year-old. If you are beginning to feel increasingly drained (physically, emotionally, and perhaps nutritionally), then the needs of your pre-born baby come before the desires of your two-year-old. Some toddlers actually increase their frequency of nursing and overall demands on their pregnant mothers because they sense something is different. Others wean toward the end of a pregnancy because the flavor of the mother's milk develops a less desirable taste. Our daughter Hayden, while still a high-need, nursing three-year-old, exclaimed toward the end of my pregnancy with her sibling, "Mommy, I don't like your milk anymore. I'll wait until after the baby comes when it is good again." You can also expect your nipples to become particularly sensitive during your pregnancy, so much so that you may no longer enjoy nursing your toddler and may need to find alternative means of comforting her. Remember, the word *nursing* implies comforting, not only breastfeeding.

57. *We have a lovely three-month-old son whom I am breastfeeding. The problem is our two-year-old, who still wants to nurse occasionally. I simply cannot handle two nursing babies. How can I get our two-year-old completely off the breast?*

Although some mothers and babies enjoy this situation (called tandem nursing), many mothers find it too exhausting. Parenting babies who are close in age is one big juggling act. One of the most frustrating feelings for dedicated parents is the realistic fact that you cannot be everything to both children at all times. A compromise is necessary. Here are some weaning tips for your particular situation:

Your two-year-old is probably fairly verbal now. Chances are, like most toddlers, he understands a good deal of what you say to him. Start negotiating, saying things such as "You can nurse, but only when the sun comes up and goes to bed." (These are favorite nursing times for toddlers and generally the last ones to be given up without a fight.) Also, since your toddler probably goes to bed and gets up at different times from your new baby, these should not be competing feeding times. Do not expect your two-year-old to say, "Okay, I'll give up this milk for the new baby." They just don't do that. Think of the nursing relationship as cutting a deep groove in your toddler's memory record. Nursing has been his most important relationship with you for two years, and he is unlikely to step aside and let someone else fill this groove. You may have heard the term *baby-led weaning*. That's a nice term, but in circumstances such as yours it is impractical. Take charge of your toddler, since this is part of disciplining him. You may say, "When you were a little baby you got a lot of Mommy's milk. Now our new baby needs a lot of Mommy's milk just like you did. You are getting older and you don't need as much of Mommy's milk."

Remember that weaning implies substituting one form of nourishment with another. When you see your two-year-old getting that "I want to nurse" look in his eye, divert his attention to another activity such as playing with a favorite toy, reading a book, or going outside to play. One-on-one activities with you will reassure him that he is still important to you. Try to avoid getting him in the cozy situations that inevitably lead to nursing. Divert him *before* he climbs up onto your lap and makes nursing overtures, or else tantrum-like behavior is likely to result.

Enlist your husband's help. Dad can remind your two-year-old that there are fun activities he can enjoy that the baby is too little for. Clue your husband in to those "about to pounce" nursing signs the older child exhibits when the new baby is being fed so that he can quickly divert your toddler's attention. You want your two-year-old to feel that he has not just lost a relationship, but has gained a new one, with his father.

58. *Our one-month-old seems to be getting colicky and gassy. I thought breastfed babies didn't get colic. Could it be some of the foods I am eating?*

Breastfed babies do get colicky, although not as often as formula-fed babies. Although it is hard to imagine scientifically that gassy foods that you eat cause gas in your baby, experience has shown that this does happen. The usual gas-producing foods are raw vegetables such as broccoli, green peppers, brussel sprouts, cauliflower, and onions. Caffeine-containing foods (colas, chocolate, coffee, and tea) may also upset your baby, although quite a large amount of these foods is usually required to bother a baby. New research has shown that dairy products are among the most common colic-producing foods in a breastfeeding mother's diet. The allergen in dairy products can pass through your milk and upset your baby. Some mothers have suspected their prenatal vitamins as causing colic in their babies. Wheat-containing foods have also been implicated in upsetting breastfeeding babies.

Some babies are highly intolerant to one or more of these foods, others may react only if their mother ingests a large quantity. The time between your ingestion of a food and the time the baby is bothered varies considerably from mother to mother. It may be as early as two hours or as late as twenty-four. In our experience babies usually show symptoms (colic, bloating, crying, rash, vomiting) within a few hours after their mothers eat the offending food. As for taking medicines while breastfeeding, it is interesting that there are actually few medicines that are harmful to the baby if taken by the breastfeeding mother. Check with a physician or health care professional who is knowledgeable about drugs and breast milk before taking a medication while breastfeeding.

If you suspect your diet, here's how you can detect the offending foods your baby may be sensitive to. Keep a diary. Eliminate the most suspicious food from your diet, beginning with dairy products, for a period of two weeks. If you notice the baby's colicy behavior lessens, reintroduce a challenge with the food eliminated. If the symptoms recur, this food goes on your no-no list. Remember, in most mother-infant breastfeeding pairs, what the mother eats does not upset the baby.

59. *My baby doesn't seem to latch on to my breasts properly. She's not getting enough milk, and I'm getting sore. What can I do to get her to breastfeed correctly?*

Proper positioning and latch-on techniques are the keys to enjoyable breastfeeding. One of the most common causes of improper latch-on is a baby not opening her mouth wide enough. Using your nipple as a teaser, gently tickle your baby's lips with your milk-moistened nipple, encouraging her to open her mouth widely. Babies' mouths can open like little birds' beaks—very wide—and then close quickly. The moment your baby opens her mouth wide, direct your nipple into her mouth and try to get as much of your areola into her mouth as possible. Remember, the milk sinuses, the reservoirs that contain the milk, are located beneath the areola of the breast so that pressure over the sinuses is necessary to squeeze out the milk. Sucking on the nipple and not the areola yields insufficient milk and leads to sore nipples.

Another common cause of improper latch-on is the position of your baby's lower lip. (When teaching interns in the hospital to counsel the breastfeeding mother, we make "lower lip rounds") Take your finger and depress your baby's lower jaw while she is latched on. This should automatically evert the lower lip, improve the seal, and eliminate that pinching feeling. If you cannot see your baby's lower lip during breastfeeding, have your husband or a trusted breastfeeding helper evert baby's lip and press down on the baby's jaw as you latch on. If you are still having difficulty after trying these techniques to improve your baby's latch-on, seek professional help from a lactation consultant. (See Appendix page 280 for breastfeeding resources.)

60. *I'm planning to return to work part-time (about thirty hours a week) two months after our expected baby is born. How should I gear up for this?*

After counseling many mothers returning to work, we have found that there are some things you can gear up for and some things you can't. Plan ahead for such things as schedules and baby-sitters and all the logistics that go into substitute mothering. Then, during the first month after your baby's birth, "forget" that you have to return to work. We have found that many mothers are so preoccupied with the future that they do not fully enjoy the present. Some mothers may feel that subconsciously they do not want to get too close to their baby because they know it will be hard to later leave him. Guard against these emotions. You are bound to experience difficulty leaving your baby anyway. Enjoy full-time mothering while you can.

61. *My wife seems absolutely addicted to our baby. She carries him all the time, sleeps with him, and generally*

*seems hooked on mothering. We have a good marriage. I
don't feel left out, and our baby seems happy, but I am
feeling pressure from colleagues at work and friends that
my wife is spoiling our baby. Could this be true?*

Your wife does seem addicted to your baby, but we use the
term addiction in a positive sense. When a mother adopts a
style of mothering which we call *attachment parenting*, the
baby does good things for a mother. Frequent nursing and
touching stimulates the hormone prolactin to come into your
wife's blood. Mothers have often confided in us that they do
feel addicted to their baby. They feel right when they are
with their baby and not right when they are separated. We
feel that this is a normal biological maternal feeling, adapted
for the development of the mother and the survival of the
baby.

    Because of peer pressure from your friends or hers,
even the most attached mother may periodically feel her
confidence in her mothering lessen. It is very important for
you to support her mothering, giving her messages that
say, "You're doing the most important job in the world—
mothering our child."

62. *Our three-month-old is developing an annoying nursing
habit. She nurses for a few minutes, pulls away for another
few, and then comes back on for a few more. Her nursing
periods during the day are growing shorter, but they are
getting longer at night. What's going on?*

This is a common nursing nuisance around three or four
months of age. It is mainly due to the rapid development of
your baby's visual acuity. She is probably able to see things
very clearly across the room and notices passersby. She is so
distracted by all the activity in her increasingly interesting
environment that she pauses frequently to attend to something visually appealing. Experienced breastfeeding mothers
have handled this nursing nuisance by "shelter nursing."
Several times a day, take your baby into a dark, quiet,

uninteresting room and get down to the business of nursing. Make the most of the pre-naptime nursing, as naptimes are usually times when the baby is more interested in her immediate environment than the world at large. Swaddling your baby will keep her limbs from swinging during nursing. Wearing your baby in a sling-type carrier and pulling the sling up over her during nursing will keep the distracted nurser from flinging her head back to explore her environment and taking your breast with her. This is a passing nursing nuisance which the above creative feeding techniques and a sense of humor will solve.

63. *I want to take off weight faster than I am now and regain my pre-pregnancy figure. What diet can I go on to lose weight but not short-change my nursing baby?*

It normally takes nine months for a lactating mother to return to her pre-pregnancy weight. Try to maintain a well-balanced diet similar to your diet during pregnancy. Avoid junk foods which are high in calories and low in nutrition. Avoid crash diets, for they are not healthy for either a nursing mother or the baby. Exercise is the safest way for a lactating mother to control her weight. One hour of sustained exercise every day, such as walking while carrying your baby, will burn off approximately three hundred calories a day. Cutting out several pieces of junk food each day will eliminate another two hundred calories from your diet, without interfering with your nutritional needs. Burning off in excess of five hundred calories a day should cause you to lose around a pound a week—a safe amount for most breastfeeding mothers. Naturally, this will depend a lot on your body type, metabolism, and how much weight you gained during pregnancy.

64. *I am trying to schedule our two-month-old breastfeeding baby, but he's not buying it. How often and for how long should I feed him?*

Early in your breastfeeding relationship you will realize that the idea of a schedule has little meaning to a breastfeeding baby. We like to replace schedule with the term harmony. Breastfeeding is more than a mathematical exercise. One nursing mother put it this way: "I don't count the number of feedings any more than I count the number of kisses." One of the most beautiful and natural biological negotiations is a mother and her nursing baby working together to get their biological clocks synchronized and the law of supply and demand working comfortably. We also wish to replace the term *demand feeding* with *cue-feeding*. This implies that you learn to read and respond to your baby's cues before he has to demand. Listen to his cues and watch him, not the clock. Remember, it is the frequency of nursing more than the duration that stimulates your milk-producing hormones. Breastfeeding cannot be scheduled easily because babies digest breast milk more rapidly than formula. Breastfed babies feel hungry more often and need to be fed more often. Tiny babies have tiny tummies. Your baby probably has frequent growth spurts during which he needs more food for more growth. Babies also enjoy periods of extra-nutritive sucking in which they are more interested in the feel than the food.

65. *My nipples are becoming quite sore. How should I care for them? Should I nurse our daughter less frequently?*

Nursing too frequently seldom causes sore nipples. The technique of nursing rather than the frequency is usually what leads to sore nipples. Teaching your baby to latch on to your areola correctly is the best preventative medicine for sore nipples. At the first sign of nipple soreness, scrutinize your technique of positioning and latch-on to be sure you are not letting the baby apply most of the pressure to your nipples rather than to your areola. Be sure your nipples are dry at all times when you're not nursing. Use fresh nursing pads, without plastic liners, to be sure no moisture is in contact with your tender skin. Let your nipples dry thoroughly before you put your bra flap up. It may be necessary to air your nipples for a while before closing your bra. If you're in a hurry, try using a blow-dryer to speed this process. A pure vegetable oil (or vitamin E from capsule, sparingly) to which neither the mother nor baby is allergic, completely massaged into the nipples after nursing, can provide local soothing and healing. A pure vegetable oil will be absorbed into the skin of your areola before the next nursing so that you do not have to wash it off. Do not use oils or creams that need to be washed off before nursing. Avoid using soap on your nipples since it may encourage dryness and cracking and remove the natural cleansing and lubricating oils.

If your nipples are getting sore from your baby clamping down too hard, pull down her lower jaw slightly during sucking, pull her closer into your breast during nursing, and nurse her in different positions so that she does not apply the same pressure at the same points on your nipple all the time. If your nipple soreness continues even after following these steps, consult a lactation specialist.

66. *My baby is three months old and I'm planning to go back to work in a couple of weeks; however, he won't take a bottle from me, whether it's my own pumped milk or infant formula. What should I do?*

During three months of breastfeeding you and your baby have set up a pattern of feeding that he has grown to anticipate. In the first few months babies set up strong patterns of association. Hunger or distress implies being picked up and breastfed. These patterns of assocation are especially deep-rooted with pleasant associations from the overall ambiance of breastfeeding. Some babies, on the other hand, will readily accept alternatives.

Try the following. Let your substitute care giver become the bottle feeder and continue to breastfeed your baby when you are with him. This causes less confusion in your baby's mind, since he continues to associate you with breastfeeding.

If you encounter a situation in which you must use a bottle, attempt to duplicate the whole environment of breastfeeding during the use of the bottle. Encourage skin-to-skin contact during the feeding and wear a short-sleeved blouse, allowing the skin of your arms to touch the skin of your baby. Engage your baby in eye-to-eye contact and try to handle him during bottle feeding the same way you do during breastfeeding.

67. *My wife is returning to work and our six-month-old daughter enjoys breastfeeding so much that she won't take a bottle from me. It is very frustrating when she is hungry and upset and I don't have the means to comfort her. What can I do?*

Shortly after this call, another father in a similar situation responded on our radio program offering the following advice: "I'm a policeman and I enjoy feeding our baby while my wife's at work. I take my shirt off and let her nuzzle against my fuzzy chest. I then hold the bottle under my arm like I'm used to holding my flashlight while I walk the beat. I hold the baby very much like my wife does at the breast while the baby nurses at the bottle held between my upper arm and chest. We both seem to get a kick out of this innovation." Hooray for a father's intuition!

68. *My baby is three months old and already I've had three breast infections. I love breastfeeding her, but these infections really drag me down. I don't want to quit breastfeeding, but how can I stop these infections?*

Usually recurrent breast infection, or mastitis, is due to some tampering with the natural law of supply and demand of breastfeeding. The natural principle of the human body is that fluid that becomes trapped anywhere in the body will become infected. Anything which lessens the emptying of your breasts or causes you to produce more than your baby consumes is a setup for breast infections. Try the following:

Review your techniques of proper latch-on. Be sure the baby has a good seal so that she empties your breast with each feeding. If your breasts still feel full after nursing, pump your excess milk either manually or with a breast pump. Try not to go too long between feedings. If your breasts "say" that it is time to feed but your baby is sleeping, either wake up your baby to feed or pump your breasts. You may have to initiate some type of regular three-hour feeding schedule during the day and once or twice at night. By keeping your breast as empty as possible, your breast infection should subside. If not, seek help from a lactation specialist to determine *why* you are having them. Some other causes include underwire bras, baby-carrier straps, strenuous upper arm exercise: i.e., jump rope or lawn mowing.

Mild breast inflammations, if treated early, easily subside by applying warm compresses and emptying the breasts. A more severe infection—fever, chills, progressive pain and tenderness—requires antibiotics. Many nursing mother wrongly think they have the flan (fatigue, fever, general aches) when in reality they have mastitis. It is rarely necessary—it may even delay healing—to stop nursing from the infected breast. If the infection is severe, pump the milk from the infected breast and allow the baby to feed from the uninfected breast.

69. *I have a problem with too much milk and my breasts become painfully engorged very easily. How can I keep this from happening?*

As in question 68, engorgement in the early weeks usually means that the basic principles of successful breastfeeding have been tampered with. Engorgement in the later months is usually due to some temporary upset in the baby's or family's routine that throws the schedule out of balance, such as trips, too many demanding visitors, or missed feedings. Engorgement is a very uncomfortable cycle. If your breasts are engorged, the nipple–areolar angle flattens so that your baby cannot suck on your areola and thus drain the underlying milk sinuses. He can only suck on a nubbin of your nipple. He gets less milk by only sucking on your nipple, but the continued sucking stimulates you to produce more milk and increases your engorgement. You keep producing but not emptying. Try the following: Pump enough of your milk to soften your breasts before feeding your baby. In this way your areolar area is softer, allowing him to latch on better and compress the milk sinuses and thus better empty your breast. A hot shower or warm towel on your breasts often stimulates the milk-ejection reflex and relieves the engorgement by releasing some milk. Try this between feedings if your baby is not ready to feed or right before a feeding to prepare your breasts.

Engorgement is both uncomfortable for the mother and frustrating for the baby. Keep your breasts as soft as you can. By keeping your breasts soft, your baby is better able to latch on and empty your breast, and you will be less prone to engorgement.

Mothers who continually have an oversupply of milk are better off using only one breast per feeding so that the breasts get completely emptied regularly and so that the sucking stimulation to each breast is decreased.

70. *With our first baby my milk suddenly came in on the fourth day and my breasts got so engorged that my baby couldn't get any milk. We're expecting another baby soon. How can I prevent this from happening again?*

As colostrum changes to milk, the quantity increases between the second and fourth day. In some mothers it happens more quickly than in others. You can minimize the engorgement resulting from your milk building up by teaching your baby correct latch-on techniques in the first few days when your breasts are still soft. If you teach your baby to get much of your areola into her mouth during this period, and she is put to breast early and often, there will be a more gradual transition to the event of breast filling. She will already have learned correct latch on and will not have to struggle with a sudden onslaught of milk. Keep your baby with you and feed as often as you can in those first few days. In our experience, engorgement occurs much less frequently in mothers who room in with their babies.

71. *Our six-month-old baby has refused to nurse the past couple of days. He is teething and just over a cold. Could this be a sign that he is ready to wean?*

This sounds more like a nursing strike. Sometime between six and twelve months some babies temporarily lose interest in nursing for a few days, and this may be erroneously interpreted as time for weaning. The cause of this temporary lack of interest in breastfeeding is usually a physical upset such as a cold or teething or some emotional upset such as a reaction to a recent change in your baby's environment or your behavior.

Here's how to entice your baby to resume nursing: For the next few days temporarily shelve all activities which drain your time and energy away from your baby. Soak in the tub together. Snuggle up in a rocking chair or sofa and cuddle and nurse as often as you can. Nap-nurse and try sleeping with your baby. (Babies often nurse in their sleep as a first step back from a strike.) By recreating the less busy, warm, and cuddly environment that he had during the first six months and by minimizing the distractions to your baby and to yourself, you recreate the nursing environment that he once knew. Thus, your baby will click in to nursing again.

72. *One of my best friends smokes a lot and is breastfeeding her baby. She doesn't smoke around the baby, but can anything from the cigarettes pass into her milk and harm her nursing infant?*

As a caring friend, try to discourage her from smoking while breastfeeding. There is some evidence that nicotine does pass into the mother's milk and therefore pass directly to the baby. Nicotine may give baby colicky symptoms. Theoretically, it could lessen the baby's growth. New studies have shown that cigarette smoking may suppress the hormone prolactin in the mother, thereby decreasing her milk supply and ability to mother. A new mother needs all the help she can get from this mothering hormone. Anything which suppresses it should definitely be discouraged.

73. *I have a happy, healthy, thriving six-month-old breast-feeding baby. Is it necessary to give her vitamin supplements?*

Unless instructed by your doctor, vitamin supplements are generally unnecessary in a healthy breastfeeding infant of a well-nourished mother. Human milk contains adequate quantities of all essential vitamins. There is still some question about the adequacy of Vitamin D in breast milk. If your diet is suspected to be low in Vitamin D or if you live in an area where exposure to sunlight is limited, especially during the winter months, Vitamin D supplements may be necessary for your baby.

74. *My friend, who is bottle feeding her baby, uses an iron-fortified formula. I am breastfeeding. Should I give our baby an iron supplement?*

Just like vitamins, breast milk contains adequate sources of iron for at least the first six to nine months of breastfeeding. You may still read occasionally that breast milk is low in iron. While breast milk *is* low in iron on paper, breast milk iron is unique in that between fifty and seventy-five percent of it is absorbed. Commercial iron may be only ten percent absorbed.

Premature babies may need iron supplements for the first few months. Around nine months, have your doctor check your baby's hemoglobin. If it is normal and your baby is starting to eat some iron-rich foods, iron supplements are not necessary.

75. *I've heard that breastfeeding may lower a woman's risk of developing breast cancer. Is this true?*

Yes. Studies have shown that women who breastfeed have a lower incidence of breast cancer. Newer studies have shown even more exciting results. The longer a mother breastfeeds, the lower her risk of developing breast cancer. In a recent study from Yale University, mothers who breastfed their infants for two years or longer had the lowest incidence of breast cancer. This is another example of the mutual benefits for a breastfeeding mother and her baby—when a mother gives something good to her baby, he gives something good back to her.

76. *Our four-month-old daughter is breastfeeding and appears fat. I thought that breastfed infants are less likely to become obese. Is this true? Also, are breastfed infants less likely to be obese children than formula-fed infants?*

In general, breastfed babies seldom become obese. It is true that some babies, especially frequent nursers, appear obese during the first six months, but in our experience this apparent extra fat inevitably disappears between six months and two years. The reason that your infant is unlikely to continue to appear obese is that breast milk undergoes exciting changes as the baby gets older. Around six months of age the fat content (and therefore the number of calories) of breast milk decreases. With increasing age infants need fewer calories per unit weight. Also, the fat of a breastfeeding baby is different than that of a formula-fed baby. Researchers have had difficulty measuring the fat in a breastfed baby because there seems to be less demarcation between fat and muscle in a breastfeeding baby, which gives a breastfeeding baby a more solid feel, even if she appears obese.

Whether breastfed infants are less likely to become obese than formula-fed infants is a subject of controversy. One can pluck from the overstuffed medical literature any study which supports one's bias. One factor about breast milk that compels me to believe that it contributes to appetite control is that breast milk changes to accommodate the needs of the infant, whereas formula does not. The fat content of breast milk changes during each feeding and also at different periods during the day. At the beginning of a nursing meal an infant sucks to get the milk flowing and obtains a large volume of foremilk (the early milk which is rich in protein and carbohydrates but low in calories). As the meal progresses, her efforts are rewarded with the richer hindmilk, which contains more fat and calories. The hindmilk may signal to her that she is full and she stops eating, having had both her sucking needs and her appetite completely satisfied. An infant may suck differently when hungry than when thirsty. When thirsty, she may only receive the lower-calorie and more watery foremilk. Formula-fed babies, however, receive the same high-calorie milk whether they are sucking for hunger or for thirst. (See question 172.)

77. *I've heard that certain herbs can increase my breast milk supply. Which ones do you recommend?*

Natural herbs which allegedly increase breast milk production are called galactogogues. Every culture has their favorite milk-enhancing potions, most of which are passed down through tradition and have not undergone any scientific analysis showing that they really do work. In our experience most mothers have found that fenugreek tea increases their milk supply. Other mothers have reported that brewer's yeast increases their milk. Some mothers, however, get quite gassy from brewer's yeast, so I'd proceed with caution.

78. *I am sick with the flu. Can I safely breastfeed my baby? Will my germs pass into my milk?*

Yes, you can breastfeed and you should. If you are coughing and sneezing, wear a mask while caring for your baby and when breastfeeding. Exciting things are going on in your milk to help protect your baby from these germs. When a germ enters your system, you make antibodies to these germs. These antibodies enter your breast milk and are then given to your baby during feeding. He then has antibodies against many of the germs that you are exposed to or that are in your system. The transfer of antibodies from a mother's milk and the degree to which they protect a baby is still a subject of research, but there does seem to be some antibody transfer. Because of the natural infection-protective properties of breast milk, it is usually safe to breastfeed your baby even though you are ill.

79. *My baby has a bad cold, and my mother-in-law says I shouldn't breastfeed her now since milk increases mucus. Is this true?*

You can safely give your baby *your* milk during a cold. Your mother-in-law is right. Milk increases mucus—cow's milk, that is. I read a recent article in a sports-medicine journal showing that cow's milk and other dairy products do in fact increase the mucus of the respiratory tract. This is probably because of the potentially allergic nature of the proteins of the cow's milk. Human babies are not allergic to the proteins in human milk, however. Go right ahead and breastfeed your baby.

80. *My baby has diarrhea and I've heard that you have to stop feeding the baby any milk while he has it. Should I stop breastfeeding until the diarrhea is cleared?*

No, unless advised to do so by your doctor. It is true that cow's milk and formula must be temporarily stopped during infections of the intestines which cause diarrhea. The reason is that the lining of the intestines is damaged by viral infections. Since this lining contains the enzymes which normally digest milk products, these products cannot be fully digested when the lining of the intestines is injured by an infection. Human milk, however, contains its own enzymes, is not a foreign protein, and is usually digested even by inflamed intestines. This is why you can usually safely breastfeed during an intestinal illness. In fact, breastfeeding has kept many babies with diarrhea out of the hospital. Because you can safely breastfeed during a diarrhea illness, the baby becomes less dehydrated and does not need to go into the hospital to have this dehydration treated as often as a baby who is being fed cow's milk or formula.

81. *I have a two-and-a-half-week-old daughter, and I'm nursing her whenever she wants it. Is it possible to overfeed her?*

It is very hard to overfeed a breast-feeding baby, and babies normally feed a lot during the first few weeks. Researchers who have studied feeding patterns in cultures that are not as schedule-oriented as we are have found that babies often feed every one to two hours around the clock during the first two weeks. Tiny babies have tiny tummies and breast milk is quickly digested. If your baby is thriving well and you are not overly tired, we advise you to go along with your newborn's feeding pattern. As your baby gets older, the intervals between feedings will lengthen.

82. *I am breastfeeding our two-week-old and we're doing well. Should I be giving him extra water?*

No, unless advised so by your doctor. Your milk is very high in water content, about ninety percent water. Breast-fed babies seldom need extra water. Studies have shown that even breastfeeding babies who live in tropical climates do not need extra water. Formula-fed babies, on the other hand, should have extra water because formula is more concentrated than breast milk. The extra water lessens the load of the more concentrated formula on your newborn's immature kidneys.

83. *My breasts have changed so much during breastfeeding. Will they ever be the same as before I started breastfeeding?*

Your breasts will never be the same as they were before your *pregnancy*. That is what made those changes, not the breastfeeding. Your pregnancy caused the growth of the milk ducts and glandular tissue. As your baby weans, your breasts will gradually return to a non-lactating state, but they will never be the same firm, totally upright shape that they were before you were pregnant. You now have the mature figure of a mother.

84. *We have an eighteen-month-old son and a two-and-a-half-month-old daughter. As soon as I sit down to nurse our baby, the older child does things he knows he's not supposed to. How can I deal with his deliberate naughtiness during those times I'm nursing our new baby?*

This is a common ploy of toddlers when they see a new baby coming into the house, getting all the attention, getting all the milk, and getting the snuggly relationship that they used to have. Undesirable behavior often occurs just at the time you are nursing the younger one. Here is a tip that we have learned from experienced moms who have lots of children and have learned to juggle to meet the needs of two children at the same time. Put together a *nursing station*. This is an area in your home where you spend the most time. It can be a family room, living room, or any other room. The nursing station should consist of the following: a rocking chair and footstool (or a comfortable pallet on the floor), pillows, a table with some nutritious snacks and water on it for you *and* your toddler, a basket of your toddler's favorite toys right next to you, a couple of your toddler's favorite books, tapes and a tape player. Reserve these books and toys and activities only for the nursing time so that your eighteen-month-old learns that nursing time for baby is also a special time for him. Instead of your toddler starting up undesirable behavior as he sees you sit down to nurse, he may now feel, "Mom does special things with me that she doesn't do at any other time." If you are on the floor with him, he will get the nonverbal message that you are available to him, and you will avoid the scene of the toddler begging to climb up in your lap just so he can be close.

85. *Our baby is two weeks old and seems to be well, but how can I be sure he's getting enough milk?*

After the first month or two you will intuitively know that your baby is getting enough milk. She will feel and look heavier. In the first few weeks it is not easy to tell if your baby is getting enough milk, especially if you are a first-time mother. Here are some signs to look for that show she is getting enough milk in the first few weeks: She wets diapers often, at least six to eight wet cloth diapers (four to five paper diapers) and two or more bowel movements per day. The character of these bowel movements gives you a clue that she is getting enough milk—the normal stool of a breastfed baby should assume a yellow mustard consistency. Also, your breasts may feel full before feedings, less full after feedings, and leak between feedings. This is also a sign that you are producing enough milk and your baby is properly emptying your breasts. If you feel her sucking vigorously, hear her swallowing, feel your milk-ejection reflex, and then see your baby drift contentedly off to sleep, chances are she has gotten enough milk.

86. *My son is just over two and a half months old, and he does not seem to be gaining weight as fast as some of my friends' babies. However, he has gained three pounds since* *birth and my doctor doesn't seem worried. How can I tell if he is getting milk?*

Some breastfed babies show a slower weight gain than their bottle-feeding colleagues. Also, your baby's body type and temperament may affect his weight gain. If he has an ecto-morph body type (long feet, long fingers, and proportion-ately taller than he is heavy) and an active temperament, expect him to gain proportionately more in length than in weight. As long as your doctor is not worried and your baby meets any of these conditions, you do not need to worry about his weight gain.

87. *I'm a tense person. How can I relax more during nursing?*

The hormone prolactin which enters your bloodstream dur-ing nursing naturally exerts a relaxing effect. Another way to create a relaxing atmosphere during breastfeeding is to create a nursing station. This is an area in your home espe-cially set up for the nursing pair, containing your favorite chair (preferably a rocking chair with arms at a comfortable height to support your arms while holding the baby), plenty of pillows, a footstool, soothing classical music, a relaxing book, nutritious nibbles, and lots of juice and water. Take the phone off the hook or have it next to you. This station is like a nest within your home to which you can retreat with your baby so you can more easily give him the quality and quantity of time he needs. Two or three deep breaths as your baby starts to feed will help relax you and will help assure that your milk flows quickly for your baby, thereby keeping him relaxed too. Having your upper back massaged along the spine helps you release your milk.

88. *How can my husband help in breastfeeding?*

Many fathers feel left out during breastfeeding. Father does, in fact, play an extremely important role in a success-ful breastfeeding relationship. In our survey of those factors

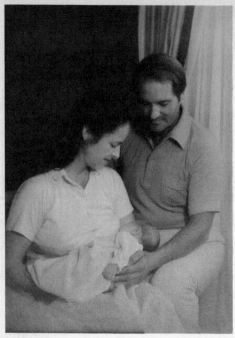

Fathers can do many things to support mothers during breastfeeding.

which contribute to successful breastfeeding, a sensitive and supportive father was high on the list. To encourage fatherly involvement it used to be advised that fathers give an occasional bottle to the baby. We do not advise this custom because of the possible interference in the law of supply and demand, the harmony, and the synchrony which occurs between mother and baby. What works better and is more biologically sound is for the father to feed the baby indirectly by improving the care and feeding of the mother. One father in a successful breastfeeding family summed it up wisely: "I can't breastfeed our baby, but I can create an environment which helps my wife breastfeed better." Fathers can bathe, walk, play with, and help with a baby (changing, burping, soothing, etc.). Breastfeeding is indeed a family affair.

89. *Our three-week-old baby doesn't seem to be gaining weight as fast as she should, and I don't feel I have enough milk. How can I increase my milk supply?*

In addition to consulting your doctor, go through the following checklist:

1. Temporarily shelve all other commitments that drain your energy from achieving harmony with your baby.

2. Avoid negative advisers who say things like, "Are you sure she's getting enough milk?" or "I couldn't breast-feed either." You don't need discouragement when you're trying to build up confidence as a new mother. Surround yourself with both supportive people and mothering organizations such as La Leche League International.

3. Take your baby to bed with you and nurse nestled close to each other. Nap nursing and night nursing are powerful stimulators for milk production, since the milk-producing hormones are best secreted while asleep.

4. Increase the frequency of feedings to at least one feeding every two to three hours, and wake your baby during the day if she sleeps more than three hours. Even a sleepy baby will nestle against your breast and stimulate your milk.

5. While you are nursing, look at and caress your baby. These maternal behaviors stimulate the milk-producing hormone.

6. Sleep when your baby sleeps. This requires delaying or delegating many seemingly pressing household chores. If you are blessed with a baby who nurses frequently, you may think, "I don't get anything done." But in fact you are doing the most important job in the world— mothering a human being.

7. Undress your baby during nursing, unless she is small (under eight pounds), in which case you need to keep the baby warm with a blanket around her, but still allowing tummy-to-tummy contact. Skin-to-skin contact may awaken sleepy babies and stimulate less enthusiastic nursers.

8. Try *switch nursing*. In the traditional method of nursing you encourage your baby to nurse as long as she wishes on one breast (usually fifteen to twenty minutes) and to

complete her feeding on the second breast, reversing the process at the next feeding. Switch nursing, also called the burp-and-switch technique, operates as follows. Let your baby nurse on the first breast until the intensity of her suck and swallow diminishes and her eyes start to close (usually three to five minutes). Remove her from this breast and burp her well; then, switch to the next breast until her sucking diminishes again; stop, burp her a second time, and repeat the entire process several times. The burp-and-switch technique encourages a creamier, high-calorie milk to come into your breast at each feeding. This technique is particularly effective for the sleepy baby, the "slurper-snoozer" who does not nurse enthusiastically.

9. Try double nursing. This technique operates on the same principle of increasing the volume and fat content of your milk as switch nursing. After you nurse your baby and she seems content, carry her around in a baby carrier instead of immediately putting her down to sleep. Burp her well and about ten to twenty minutes later, breastfeed her a second time. Keeping the baby upright for ten to twenty minutes following the feeding allows the trapped bubble of air to be burped up, leaving room for a topping-off with more milk.

10. Get support from breastfeeding organizations such as La Leche League International. This network of professional mothers can provide you with the support you need during those confusing first few months. Breastfeeding requires confidence. A good support group will help you develop this confidence.

If you are still having trouble with your milk supply after trying the above suggestions, don't give up. See a lactation specialist.

90. *Our baby is three months old and I am returning to full-time work, but I don't want to stop breastfeeding. Can I continue? How?*

Yes, you can and we advise you to. Here are some tips that we give in our breastfeeding clinic to help mothers continue breastfeeding when returning to work.

1. Purchase a (battery-operated or plug-in) portable breast pump. While at work, take frequent breaks to pump your milk, at least every three hours. (Incidentally, you have a legal right to this time off to pump your milk.) Store this milk in a clean bottle in a refrigerator or iced cooler and take it home to the baby-sitter to be used the following day or freeze it for future use.

2. Breastfeed your baby before you leave for work in the morning, as soon as you return home in the afternoon, throughout the evening, and as frequently as possible during weekends and holidays. The "happy departure" nursing (before leaving for work in the morning) and the "happy reunion" nursing (upon returning home in the evening) are usually the most pleasant.

3. Encourage your substitute care giver to give your baby a late-afternoon nap and to avoid feeding him within an hour before you're expected home. As soon as you return home, take the phone off the hook, turn on some soothing music, put your feet up, and nurse. Many mothers find that breastfeeding their baby as soon as they return home helps them unwind from a hectic day's work. This is probably due to the relaxing effect of the hormone prolactin, which mothers describe as better and certainly healthier than the after-work cocktail.

4. Share sleep with your baby. Many mothers report that upon returning to work their baby begins to wake up frequently. They are so tired from being up and down with their baby all night that they find it difficult to work the next day. The reason for this is that babies often tune out the baby-sitter during the day and become frequent night feeders. This nuisance can be alleviated by allowing your baby to sleep next to you so that neither you nor your baby fully awakens during feeding and your sleep is

therefore less disturbed. Night nursing also allows your milk supply to continue.

5. Encourage or, better yet, insist that your husband do his share of household chores. If you are going to continue breastfeeding and working, you need domestic help.
6. Think "baby" while at work. Many mothers instinctively surround themselves with pictures of their baby while at their office. It also helps to have a picture (both actual and mental) of your baby while using the breast pump. This helps activate your milk-producing hormones.
7. Be prepared for temporary adjustment nuisances, such as engorgement or leaking. These discomforts will subside within a few weeks as your body adjusts to your new breastfeeding routine.
8. Further tips on breastfeeding and working can be obtained from your local chapter of La Leche League International.

91. *Another breastfeeding mother and I share baby-sitting. Sometimes when I am late getting back and my baby is upset, she will have breastfed her. Is this all right?*

Breastfeeding organizations that we have interviewed on this subject generally discourage the practice of substitute breastfeeding, perhaps because they feel that since breastfeeding is such a special relationship, it may confuse the baby to switch back and forth. We feel that substitute breastfeeding in emergency circumstances is all right providing you know this mother well and that she and her baby are free of infections. The fact that your friend is willing to do this implies that she is a nurturing person. Whatever you decide about the substitute breastfeeding, treasure her as a friend.

92. *My baby is a gulper during nursing and swallows a lot of air. He is difficult to burp. Any suggestions?*

Be sure your baby is getting mostly milk at each feeding and not a lot of air. Some eager feeders are so anxious to eat that they seem to hyperventilate for a few seconds in anticipation of feeding. Try to anticipate your baby's feeding cues more quickly and feed him before he becomes too anxious and begins to breathe rapidly. Examine the seal of your baby's mouth on your breast. The position of the lips is the key. Be sure your baby's lips are turned outward. The lower lip is sometimes difficult to observe during feeding. Ask your husband to evert your baby's lower lip during feeding for this will give a more airtight seal.

In addition, here are some burping suggestions: Burp your baby at least once during the feeding (usually when switching breasts) in addition to after the feeding. Remember, effective burping techniques require both an upright position and pressure on the abdomen. Lean your baby's weight against the heel of your hand as he sits on your lap, or drape him over your shoulder or over one knee, and firmly pat or rub his back. If you drape him over your shoulder or over your knee, the pressure on his tummy will help relieve his stomach of air. If you sit your baby upright on your knee, use one hand to pat his back gently and the other to press gently against his tummy just above the navel. Most parents forget that gentle pressure on the tummy is an important step in effective burping.

93. *Our six-month-old has slowed down on her nursing during the day, but awakens three or four times during the night, and I'm tired. How can I get her to nurse less during the night?*

This is a very common and exhausting feeding pattern during the second half of the first year. Babies become so busy and so easily distracted during the day that they would rather do other things than feed. They become day players and night feeders. To reverse this pattern, purposely feed your baby every two hours during the day. You may have to feed her in a dark, quiet, non-stimulating environment and fill her up on breast milk (and sucking) during the day. Soon your baby will get the idea that daytime is for eating and playing, and nighttime is for sleeping. Remember, one or two feedings at night is considered normal. And starting solids often doesn't help a baby sleep through. See question 147.

94. *We have a happy, healthy one-year-old son who is still breastfeeding. I have no great desire to wean him; however, my husband and I would like to have a second child, and have heard that nursing decreases my chances of conceiving. Can you help me solve this problem?*

It is true that frequent breastfeeding, especially night nursing, does suppress ovulation and may lessen your chances of getting pregnant again. If you wish to continue nursing yet also want to become pregnant again soon, here are some suggestions: The frequent nighttime breastfeedings are what mainly suppress ovulation. We would suggest you try weaning your child from any breastfeeding at night, but breastfeed him as needed during the day. If your one-year-old has been sharing your bedroom at night, weaning may be best accomplished by having your husband sleep with the baby for a few nights and try a father's comforting rather than breastfeeding as a means of nighttime security. After a few weeks of omitting nighttime feedings, your fertility will likely return.

You are right not to want to wean your child completely. When you have a happy, secure baby, don't do anything that might jepordize his feelings of security. (See related question 55.)

95. *Our two-year-old is still nursing. She enjoys it and so do I, but I'm getting a lot of flack from my friends. ("What! You're still nursing?") Is it all right to nurse a baby this long, and second, how do I fend off my friends?*

Mothers often ask us how long they should nurse their baby. We have a sign in our office which reads, "Early weaning not recommended for babies." It may help you to understand the real meaning of the word weaning. In ancient Hebrew writings, it meant "to ripen." The word that was used when a fruit was ripe and ready to be picked from the vine was the same as the word used for weaning. It was a positive step and wasn't associated with the end of a relationship. It represented a passage from one relationship to another. Weaning was a festive occasion because the child was now ripe and ready to take on new relationships such as the beginning of formal instruction by his father and the wise men in the town. This is why weaning occurred around the third *year*, when the child was verbal enough and had developed enough intellectual competence to begin education. A child was weaned from the security of his mother into the arms of the culture, with no break in the action.

Life is a series of weanings for a child: weaning from the womb, weaning from the breast, weaning from the parents' bed, weaning from home to school and from school to work. The age at which a child is ready to wean varies tremendously from child to child. One who is weaned from any of these stages before she is ready is at high risk of developing problems associated with premature weaning: anger, aggression, mood swings, etc. This is often why tantrum-like behavior begins in a toddler who is weaned before his time.

In our opinion, a nursing toddler is a beautiful sight. Expect raised eyebrows from poorly informed onlookers whose negative feelings toward breastfeeding betrays their lack of understanding of the toddler as a little person with big needs. For a toddler, breastfeeding is seldom a prime source of nutrition, but rather a consoling lift during periods of stress.

Here's some ammunition to fend off your critics: In our experience and that of others, one of the best investments that you can make into the physical and emotional health of your child is to not wean her before her time. The children we have studied who have nursed well into their second year or longer generally are most independent, more secure, and separate more easily from their mothers later on than children who have been weaned before their time. Extended nursing does not cause dependency; it fills a need. A need that is filled eventually goes away. A need that is not completely filled never completely goes away but manifests itself in undesirable behavior. You are right in what you are doing.

In counseling mothers who do wish to wean, we have found that timely weaning actually broadens the mother–baby interaction rather than lessens it. In some mother–infant pairs, nearly all the interaction revolves around breastfeeding—a source of nutrition, comfort, play, sleep induction, etc. After weaning, a mother will learn skills other than breastfeeding to carry on these interactions.

3

NIGHT WAKING

Night waking problems top the list of questions we are asked. Most of these questions stem from the fact that new parents often have unrealistic expectations about babies' sleep patterns. Many night waking problems occur because mother and baby are out of nighttime harmony with each other or because the right sleeping arrangements were not attempted. The answers given to the following questions are based upon what we have learned over our twenty years of parenting and an almost equal number of years in pediatric practice. They are based upon the years of personal research which we did in preparation for our book *Nighttime Parenting*. There is more erroneous advice about solutions to night waking than perhaps in any other aspect of infant care.

Everyone in the family has nighttime needs. In the following answers we have attempted a balanced approach toward meeting the needs of the entire family while at the same time respecting the fact that babies have a unique set of nighttime needs that are often unrecognized by new parents, and for that matter, by most authors of baby books.

Our goal in this chapter is to help *everyone* in the family enjoy a good night's sleep.

96. *Our three-month-old baby still wakes up one or twice at night for a feeding no matter where he sleeps, either in his own bed or in ours. He goes back to sleep easily after I feed him and so do I. However, I've read that babies are supposed to be sleeping through the night at three months. Is this true?*

Many books do proclaim that babies should be sleeping through the night at three months, but most babies have not read these books. In actual fact, the only babies who sleep through the night at three months are "everyone else's baby." The age at which babies settle down—meaning going to sleep easily and staying asleep—varies tremendously and is usually a reflection of your baby's temperament and not of your nighttime parenting skills. Keep in mind that during the first six months, or even a year for some babies, a baby wakes up easily. They do not wake up to annoy you or to purposely keep you awake. The longer we practice pediatrics and the more children we have, the more we realize that babies do what they do because they are designed that way. A thorough explanation of why babies sleep differently than adults will help you understand and therefore sympathize with your baby's frequent night waking.

Babies and adults have two different sleep patterns. For simplicity we will call these two patterns *light sleep* and *deep sleep.* During light sleep, the higher brain centers are not completely shut down and the sleeper may awaken easily. During deep sleep, the higher brain centers shut down, allowing the sleeper to drift into a very deep, almost motionless state of sleep. The main difference between adult and baby sleep is that adults spend approximately eighty percent of their night sleep in the state of deep sleep, whereas with babies the reverse is true. They spend most of the night in light sleep. This hardly seems fair to you until you realize that babies are purposely designed that way for both survival and developmental reasons. A baby has the highest percentage of light sleep during those early months when his nighttime needs are highest, but his ability to communicate them is lowest. Suppose he had a stuffy nose and could not breathe, yet couldn't easily awaken to communicate this need? Suppose he were hungry and needed food, yet did not easily awaken to cry? Suppose he was cold and did not easily awaken to signal this need for warmth? If a baby had the same predominance of deep sleep states as we do, his survival would be in jeopardy. As the baby grows older, the percentage of light sleep gradually decreases as the percentage of deep sleep increases.

Another interesting reason why babies have a large percentage of light sleep is tied to their need for developmental stimulation. Prominent sleep researchers feel that during the state of light sleep, the higher brain centers continue to function, and this functioning is necessary for the brain to mature. I was explaining this theory to a very tired mother of a frequent night waker when she exclaimed, "In that case my baby is going to be very, very smart!"

97. *Our six-month-old baby just won't go to sleep by herself. I know she's tired; she falls asleep in my arms. However, when I put her into her crib and try to tiptoe out of the room, she wakes up and screams.*

Another unrealistic expectation of nighttime parenting during the first year, and sometimes even longer, is that you can put your baby down in the crib at a preset time, pat her "night-night," and expect her to stay asleep. Although some babies do this, most don't. The reason is that babies are not designed to go to sleep the same way adults are. When we fall asleep, we can go quickly into a state of deep sleep without first passing through a long period of light sleep. Infants, however, enter a long period of light sleep before they can enter deeper sleep. This period of initial light sleep averages around twenty minutes. If an arousal stimulus such as a squeaky crib, sudden change of position (such as being put into the crib), or a disturbing noise occurs during this initial light sleep stage, the baby will reawaken easily because she has not yet reached the deep sleep state. This accounts for the fact that your baby is difficult to settle or, as some mothers say, "She has to be fully asleep before she can be put down." Some infants enter quickly into the deep sleep state by three to six months, others take longer.

You might want to try this nighttime parenting style: Lie down with your baby on your bed or any place that allows both of you to snuggle close to each other if you are breastfeeding. If you are bottle feeding, a rocking chair should suffice. Nurse (either breast or bottle) your baby until you notice that she has drifted through the state of light sleep into the state of deep sleep. You can recognize that she is still in the state of light sleep by the following signs: fluttering eyelids, facial grimaces, fists partially clenched, muscle twitches, and overall body muscle tone unrelaxed. Nurse your baby until these signs subside and she has entered a state of deep sleep, recognizable by an almost motionless face, regular respirations, still eyelids, and what we call the limp-limb signs: Her arms dangle weightlessly from her sides, her hands are open, and her overall muscles are relaxed. After your baby is in a state of deep sleep you can either put her in her crib or quietly detach yourself and sneak away. Babies will usually stay asleep once they are in this state of deep sleep. (See question 131.)

98. *Our two-month-old baby wakes up four or five times a night. I can't stand to let him cry, but by the time I get to him he's a wreck and I'm a wreck. It's taking me longer to resettle him and get back to sleep myself. My baby does not seem tired the next day, but I certainly am. Can you help?*

You and your baby are out of nighttime harmony with each other. Another difference between babies and adults is that babies have much shorter sleep cycles than adults. A sleep cycle occurs every time we go from a state of light sleep to deep sleep and back up into light sleep. In adults this cycle occurs around every two hours. In babies these sleep cycles may change every hour. Every time a person, especially a baby, goes from the state of deep sleep into the state of light sleep, he goes through a vulnerable period for night waking. Some babies wake up during these vulnerable periods, others do not. It sounds as if you have a light sleeper who wakes up each time he changes sleep cycles. The reason you are tired is that you and your baby are out of sync. He probably wakes up during his light sleep cycles while you are aroused out of your deep sleep cycles. The way a person wakes up, not the frequency of waking, causes sleep deprivation. This is the reason that you are more tired than your baby is the next day.

Here's how to reach nighttime harmony with your baby. Take him into your bed either initially or after the first night waking. Nurse him to sleep, and again whenever he wakes up. After a few nights of this you will notice that you and your baby begin to get your sleep cycles in sync with each other so that as your baby enters the state of light sleep and starts to wake up, so do you. You can then roll over and nurse your baby through his vulnerable period for night waking. You will both then drift back into the state of deep sleep without having fully awakened. And he won't wake at each cycle because just your closeness will smooth his transition from deep to light and back to deep without waking at all. He'll waken only when he needs to be fed.

Not all mother–infant pairs achieve this nighttime harmony, but if you can, it works beautifully toward getting you and your baby a good night's sleep. This is also called organizing your baby. One of our goals in early nighttime parenting is to organize our baby's sleep cycles to minimize night waking. When you and your baby achieve this nighttime harmony, you are well on your way to enjoying a better night's sleep. See also questions 126 and 127 for restless, fitful night waking.

99. *Our one-year-old is such a light sleeper that the slighest noise disturbs her. How can I keep her from waking up?*

Every baby seems to have a different stimulus threshold for night waking. Some babies could sleep through a trumpet blast, others seem to wake up at the sound of a pin dropping. Try the following tips to reduce the stimuli that usually cause night waking: Oil all moving parts on your baby's crib to prevent squeaking. If you are using cloth diapers, minimize the wetness of the diaper area by putting two diapers on your baby before bedtime. If your baby is sensitive to sudden noises, you may help her settle down by using "white noise" such as the fan of an air conditioner or running water. This noise is so repetitive and meaningless that it lulls the mind to sleep. The most effective sleep-inducing sounds for a baby are those which most closely resemble the rhythm and sounds of the womb: running water from a nearby faucet or shower; a metronome set at sixty beats per minute; a ticking clock; a recording of womb sounds; a bubbling fish tank; or a tape recording of waterfalls or ocean sounds. Find the sounds that work best to keep your baby sleeping and tape-record them. Use a recorder with automatic replay that keeps on playing. As your baby gets older and her sleep patterns mature, she will not arouse so easily.

100. *Our three-year-old wakes up early and comes into our bedroom around five-thirty every morning and wants to play. How can I get that extra hour of golden sleep in the morning?*

Here are some tips on delaying the early riser:

1. Put blackout curtains over his windows.
2. If you have older siblings, lay down rules for a noiseless awakening.
3. Give your child an alarm clock "just like Mommy's and Daddy's."
4. Leave a "surprise box" at his bedside. Each morning put

a couple of different toys in this box so that he looks forward to his morning surprise. The deal is that he has to play with them awhile before awakening you!

5. Leave a nutritious snack on a bedside table to tide over your hungry riser until breakfast.

6. He may enjoy climbing into bed with you and going back to sleep—it's worth a try!

101. *Our four-year-old wakes up in the middle of the night, comes into our bedroom, and climbs into our bed. I don't mind her coming into our room, but I don't like being awakened. Should I lock our door?*

No. This usually does not solve the problem. As long as you do not mind her joining you in the middle of the night, the key is to teach her how to do so without waking you up. Children do need to respect the fact that nighttime is for sleeping. Put a sleeping bag or a futon at the foot of your bed. Tell your daughter that if she does come in, she must go as "quietly as a mouse" directly into her special bed and stay there quietly until Mom and Daddy wake up. This gives your child the messages that you are available to her at night, but that she must respect that nighttime is for sleeping.

102. *I've recently returned to work, and our four-month-old has begun to wake up more frequently. I'm up and down all night trying to resettle him into his crib. I'm so tired that it's hard to work the next day. I need some nighttime help.*

This is a common nighttime nuisance when mothers return to work. We frequently hear the following scenario: Mother picks her baby up at the baby-sitter and the baby-sitter exclaims, "My, what a good baby. She slept all day." Babies sometimes learn to tune out the baby-sitter during the day and sleep in order to save their waking time to be with you at night. It almost seems that they are deliberately getting their days and nights mixed up. Remember that babies do what they do for a reason. Every baby has a critical need for touch time with his parents, and some need more than others. Your baby is probably telling you, "Mommy, I need more time with you." Here's how to give your baby more touch time and yourself more sleep: Take him into your bed and enjoy sleeping side by side. If you are breastfeeding, allow him to nurse at night. Because neither you nor your baby is used to this sleeping arrangement, you may need a few weeks to get accustomed to sleeping together. In our counseling of working mothers, we have found that sharing sleep is one of the best ways to get nighttime needs of the infant met while helping his mother to get a good night's sleep in order to carry on her job the next day. (See question 106.)

103. *We would like to have our new baby sleep with us, but my doctor advises us not to. I'm confused. Who is right?*

There are three questions you should not ask your doctor: "Where should my baby sleep?" "How long should my baby nurse?" and "Should I let my baby cry?" Doctors do not study the answers to these questions in medical school, and much of their advice likely comes from their own personal experience as mothers and fathers and not as professionals. You are putting doctors on the spot when you ask them where your baby should sleep. Doctors are trained in the diagnosis and treatment of illnesses, not in parenting styles. If you want to sleep with your baby and feel that your baby, your husband, and you will all sleep better with this nighttime parenting style, this is the right decision for your family.

Incidentally, you will find that in recent years doctors have become increasingly flexible about parents sleeping with their babies. Doctors are now realizing that they do not have to spend so much time counseling parents about sleep problems later on if they spend more time helping a baby create a healthy sleep attitude in the early months.

104. *We are doing a lot of reading about how to take care of our baby, who is due next month. We are intrigued with the idea of the family bed. How does it work?*

A fact of parenting is that you do a lot of juggling of sleeping arrangements during your baby's first year. Our advice is that wherever all three of you, mother, father, and baby, sleep the best is the right arrangement for you. We are glad that you are open to trying various arrangements. Openness is the key to nighttime parenting—in fact, to all of parenting. Incidentally, we prefer the term *sharing sleep* rather than the family bed, which implies a host of children all snuggled together with their parents in one bed. In our experience it often does not work to have a lot of children in one bed. The term sharing sleep implies you share more than just bed space, you share sleep cycles. We advise parents to begin sleeping with their baby right after they come home from the hospital. This allows you and your baby to harmonize your sleep cycles with each other, makes nighttime nursing easier, lessens night waking, and generally gives you and your baby that extra touch time. Your baby is probably going to wake up frequently. The key is to minimize her waking and to get her back to sleep as easily as you can, preferably without even waking up yourself. Sharing sleep helps you accomplish this.

105. *Our baby sleeps with us and we really enjoy it, but sometimes he wakes up in the middle of the night bright-eyed and bushy-tailed and ready to play. Initially this was funny, but now we're tired of it. How can I stop the habit?*

Infants need nighttime conditioning. They need to learn that a bed is for sleeping, not for playing. We have solved this nighttime nuisance in our family by "playing dead." When our eighteen-month-old wakes up eager to play, we pretend that we are still asleep and ignore his desire to play. Initially this is tough to do, since your baby will probably start to crawl all over you trying to get your attention. If you persist long enough, though, he will eventually get the message that nighttime is for sleeping and not for playing. This is not the same as letting your baby cry. Babies seldom cry to play. Intense nighttime crying usually signals a need. Your baby is secure because you are there; his wanting to play is a whim and not a need. A bit of nighttime humor is also necessary to help you survive your 3:00 A.M. playmate.

106. *I've recently gone back to work and find that I am often so tense and wide awake at night that I can't get to sleep. Other times my three-month-old daughter wakes up often, and then neither one of us can get to sleep. We both need help.*

Here is a good example of the concept of mutual giving. Take your baby to bed with you and nurse her off to sleep. Something good happens to both of you when you sleep and nurse next to each other. Researchers have recently discovered that your milk contains a sleep-inducing substance. When you give your baby your milk at night you are helping put her to sleep. The other side of the nighttime parenting equation is that when your daughter nurses from you she stimulates the hormone prolactin to enter your bloodstream. This hormone acts as a natural tranquilizer which helps to put and keep you asleep. Many working mothers have shared with us that night nursing really helps them sleep better after a tough day.

107. *Our one-year-old used to sleep very well; but now he is beginning to wake up more frequently. I go in and find him standing up in his crib as if he wants to get out. Why is he doing this and what should I do?*

Night waking frequently occurs when babies have developed a new major developmental skill, such as going from sitting to crawling (at around six to seven months) and from crawling to walking (around one year). Babies wake up and become so aware of their newfound skill that they want to practice it even at night. For the beginning walker, the confines of the crib may be somewhat restrictive. When you go in to your baby, try to resettle him with a minimum of fuss. Put a rocking chair next to his crib and try to rock him back to sleep. If you can, get him to resettle without getting him out of the crib; even better, try getting him to lie down and pat him or massage him while singing to him. Several ingenious mothers have shared with us a tip: They lower the side rail to the level of the mattress, bend over, and nurse the baby while he is still lying in the crib. This often resettles him without having to pick him up out of the crib. Night waking due to development of a new motor skill usually subsides once this skill is mastered.

108. *Our two-year-old is ready to leave our bedroom, and I'm trying to decide whether it's best to get him his own room or let him sleep with his older brother. Any suggestions?*

If your child has been accustomed to sleeping close to someone, it is unlikely that he will sleep well in his own room, even snuggled up with something like a teddy bear. Part of the normal nighttime weaning is to wean a toddler from the parents' bed into a sibling's room and then into his own room. Studies have shown that children under three sleep better sharing a bedroom rather than in their own. We have also noticed that siblings who sleep together quarrel less. Watch for your child's cues that he is ready for his own room. Most children around three years old desire some private space for their many personal belongings. A child's own room helps foster a sense of order and a sense of responsibility through caring for his belongings. Construct low-lying shelves, compartments for toys, and pegs for hanging clothes.

An additional word of advice: We do not feel that separate bedrooms are important enough to require a family to overextend themselves financially by working longer hours and further separating themselves from their children in order to afford a house with more bedrooms.

109. *Our two-year-old just doesn't seem to need a nap, but I need her to take one. Do two-year-olds need naps? How can I get her to nap so that I can get something done?*

Yes, most two-year-olds need naps; at least, their parents need them to need naps. In the first year most babies need at least a one-hour nap in the morning and a one-to-two-hour nap in the afternoon. Between one and two years some babies drop the morning nap, but still require a one-to-two-hour afternoon nap. Most children require at least a one-hour afternoon nap until around the age of four. Sleep researchers feel that napping does have restorative value. Some children and adults actually fall asleep more quickly and sleep more efficiently during a short nap than they do during the night.

Here's how to encourage your child to take a nap: Nap with her. I realize that you mentioned that this would be a time for you to get something done. Many mothers feel that way, but naps are equally as important for parents as they are for children. Even if your child doesn't want to nap, she may need a little "down time." Choose the same time of the day (a time that you're the most tired) and set your child up for a nap. Take her into a quiet room, turn on some soft music, darken the room, and nestle together in a rocking chair or lie down on a bed. Set aside a special time every day for a quiet time in which you read a story or some lulling and soothing activity. Sometimes your child chooses to sleep during this time, other times not. Be flexible about where she is allowed to nap. Some children resist going to their bedroom for a nap, but will crash for a nap somewhere else in the house. We have used a "nap nook," a special place in a corner with a soft rug or a little tent made of blankets into which the child crawls when she is tired. This technique capitalizes on children's natural desire to construct their own little retreats throughout the house. Lambskin mats are also a good place for babies to nap. We learned this trick while giving a series of parenting lectures in Australia where lambskins are plentiful. Mothers would often bring their babies to our talks, and shortly before the talk was ready to begin they placed their lambskin next to their feet and put their baby down for a nap. Babies had been conditioned to associate lambskins with napping. Whenever the lambskin was stretched out, they were set up for a nap. Be sure your baby is not allergic to wool. It helps to cover the lambskin with a cloth diaper.

110. *I often need an hour to put our three-year-old to bed. He keeps nagging, "Daddy, just one more story." I'm tired. He isn't. How can I get him to be less demanding at bedtime?*

Most bedtime procrastinators are put to bed by parents who are not around much during the day. Children quickly realize that nighttime is the only time when they may have their parents, especially fathers, all to themselves. Expect your child to try everything possible to prolong this special one-on-one time. You may survive these bedtime rituals better by appreciating how much your son really wants to spend time with you.

Here's a tip that may shorten your bedtime ritual: Lie down on the bed next to your son, with the lights out, of course. I've noticed that our children fall asleep faster when I lie down with them. This style of nighttime fathering is especially valuable if you leave for work early in the morning before your child awakens. Rather than reading a story with the lights on, a better sleep inducer is telling bedtime stories with the lights dimmed. Children love to hear homespun tales about your childhood. A back rub is another soothing way to father a child to sleep. Using the power of suggestion, tell your child that he is falling asleep as you work your hands down from his head to his feet. Reassure him that you will stay with him until he is asleep.

111. *We like music at night and so does our baby. What type of music helps babies sleep best?*

Most babies settle better with classical music than with turbulent rock music. Choose music which is simple and consistent, such as flute or classical guitar. Studies have shown that even prenatal babies are soothed better with classical music than with rock music. (As the parents of teenagers, we wonder if a child's musical taste steadily deteriorates from birth to adolescence . . . or if, perhaps, it's just a passing phase.) Music that has closely rising crescendos and decrescendos with a minimum of sudden changes in tempo usually soothes babies the best. Some researchers have reported that Brahms, Beethoven, and Bach soothe babies the best, while others disagree with these selections. In our experience Mozart and Vivaldi are at the top of the nighttime classical hit list. Select a medley of pieces that best soothe your baby and prepare your own tape from the records of these pieces. Some babies need music only to get to sleep; others need continuous music to stay asleep. We suggest a continuous-play recorder with auto-reverse to keep the music playing.

112. *We really want our baby to sleep in our room, since we have read so much about the advantages. However, she seems to wake up more when sleeping close to us, and so do I. I'm kind of disappointed that this arrangement isn't working.*

No one sleeping arrangement works for all babies all the time. Some are so sensitive that they wake up more frequently when sleeping next to their parents; likewise, some parents are particularly light sleepers. An alternative to sharing your bed is what we call the "sidecar" arrangement. Remove one side rail from your baby's crib and place this open side adjacent to your bed. Adjust the crib mattress level to the exact level of your mattress. Be sure there is no crevice between your baby's mattress and yours. This allows you and your baby to be in close nursing and touching distance to each other while allowing both of you to have your own sleeping space, which it sounds like you need.

Some babies seem to have a critical sleeping distance. Too far or too close from you increases their night waking. The sidecar is a good compromise. This arrangement also works well for families who want to try having their baby in their bed, but don't have a king-size bed or have a baby who is such a squirmer that she needs her own space.

113. *I really want to sleep with our baby, but my husband is not keen on the idea. Our baby is due soon. How can I win my husband over?*

Sharing sleep with your baby does not work well unless both the mother and father are in agreement about this sleeping arrangement. I initially had reservations about the idea of sleeping with our baby in our bed, but I gave in to my wife's strong convictions that this was right. In deed, with one of our children, that's the only way both my wife and the infant could sleep. I have since come to enjoy the closeness. I do not have as much time with my children as I want to, so nighttime gives me an opportunity to be close to our babies. I particularly enjoy waking in the morning and gazing upon the face of our "sleeping beauty" lying only a few feet or inches away. I have grown accustomed to waking up with a baby in our bed. In short, I'm hooked and I hope you can get your husband hooked too!

Here's a letter that we recently received from a mother in your situation: "Totally breastfeeding our son on demand led us to try sleeping with our baby in our bed. A big plus is not having to get out of a warm bed several times a night to feed the baby. We have fine-tuned our nursing techniques so that now neither I nor the baby fully awakens for feedings. We made a pact that my husband was to be the barometer in this relationship. In order to respect his feelings, we decided that if he thought it was not working out, we'd get a crib. Well, we don't have one yet! All three of us enjoy the closeness, and we rest secure in the knowledge that the baby is okay—warm, right next to us, and easy to find in the dark. Our baby rarely wakes up crying in the morning.

We are usually right there and he is content and happy. A nice way to start each day."

A key to this mother's solution was to allow her husband to be the barometer in this situation. If your husband does not look forward to having a baby sleep between you, here's an alternative which often works better anyway. Place your baby between you and a guardrail (a device which attaches under your mattress and flips up alongside your bed, available at baby furniture stores). Sleeping with your baby between you may keep both of you awake, since babies often turn all the way around during the night and Dad may wake up with cold feet in his back. This will not win your baby points for sleeping in your bed. If your husband is still unconvinced, encourage him to read our books *Nighttime Parenting* and *Becoming a Father.* I'm willing to wager that these books will get him interested in the idea. (See questions 103, 104, 112.)

114. *I've read a lot about the family bed. Many of my friends let their babies sleep in their beds, but quite honestly I just don't want to. We have four children, and by the time evening comes I've had enough of kids. I want some time alone with my husband. Am I wrong to feel this way?*

We support your feelings. You honestly feel that for your particular family situation, it is necessary for you to have this special time with your husband at night to nurture the marriage, recharge your own batteries, and be a more effective mother by day. This decision is not selfish but represents a realistic appraisal that the whole family would probably function better if you have separate sleeping arrangements. It sounds like you have realistic expectations of your own needs and also that you are probably blessed with a baby who is not particularly separation-sensitive at night. The best sleeping arrangement for one family may not be the best for another. Our advice is that wherever all members of the family sleep the best and feel right is the best sleeping arrangement for the family. Don't feel pressured

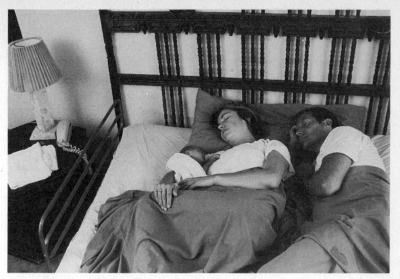

The family bed.

into a nighttime parenting style that you don't believe in simply because your friends are endorsing it.

115. *I am expecting a baby in a month, and our three-year-old is still sleeping with us. I don't want to exile her from our bed, but I honestly feel I can't handle two kids at night.*

Making room for a new baby while another child is already in your bed is indeed a difficult problem. In our experience, having more than one child in your bed at one time doesn't work. If you don't relish having both your three-year-old and your new baby in your bed, here are some alternatives: The problem is persuading your three-year-old to accept an alternative without feeling banished from her nighttime place of security. Remember, weaning a child from your bed means you must substitute alternative forms of comfort and nighttime nourishment. As you mother your newborn at night, ask your husband to father the three-year-old. Treat this as something special: "Daddy and you are going to sleep together on a big mattress . . . ," either at the foot of your bed or in your three-year-old's own room. She will probably feel that though she has lost a bit of Mommy, she has gained more of Daddy with no overall net loss. You may also try a futon or a kiddy-type sleeping bag at the foot of your bed. It might be wise to begin suggesting this alternative sleeping arrangement before your new baby comes.

116. *Our six-month-old baby used to be such a good sleeper, but now he wakes up several times a night. Could this be teething?*

Yes. Teething pain often accounts for frequent night waking in babies between five and seven months of age who previously settled down well. Although you may not actually feel or see your baby's teeth until around seven or eight months, teething discomfort may start as early as four months. Teething is accompanied by profuse drooling, and you may notice the telltale signs of a wet bed sheet under his head and a drool rash on his cheeks and chin where he has rubbed his face against the wet sheets. Teething can continue to be a cause of night waking, for additional teeth come in all the way through the two-year molars. To minimize the pain associated with teething and possibly the resultant night waking, give your baby an appropriate dose of acetaminophen before going to bed and once or twice again during the night. (The dose on the box can be increased by checking with your doctor.)

Another common reason for night waking around six months is that your baby is going through a major developmental milestone: sitting up by himself. Many times babies wake up, sit up, and then want to practice playing by sitting up and then pulling themselves up on the sides of the crib. You may need to go in and resettle him in the tummy-sleeping position.

117. *Our four-month-old has just begun to wake frequently, and squirms around a lot more at night. I'm puzzled because she used to be such a good sleeper. Any ideas?*

Around four months of age babies begin to roll over at night, usually from tummy to back. Suddenly finding herself in a different position may be unsettling to a half-awake baby. Also, she may not be able to get herself back on her tummy (like a flipped-over turtle!) and therefore cannot fall asleep on her own. You may need to turn her back over, pat her on the back, and help her resettle into her favorite sleeping position.

118. *We have a two-year-old and a six-month-old, and I can't get them to nap at the same time. When my baby takes his nap I would love to join him, but it seems like this is just the time when our older child demands time from me. I feel strung out between both of our children's demands.*

The more children you have, the sooner you will realize that parenting is a juggling act. Synchronizing siblings' naps is difficult. You can't always be all things to all of your children. Although mothers do seem to defy many laws of mathematics, you just can't give a hundred percent to each child all the time. Call in the reserves. Get your two-year-old involved in a play group for a few afternoons each week. When Dad is home, take shifts. Dad takes the older child while you nap with your baby. Set your older child up for some quiet time by turning on some records and getting him started on some quiet play. If he is confined to a safe area with easy access to you, you can lie down and doze with your baby while at the same time keeping one ear open for your two-year-old.

119. *Our baby is almost two and seems to be waking up more. I go in and find her standing up rattling the sides of her crib. Could she be ready for a regular bed?*

The age at which babies progress from crib to bed varies tremendously, but here are some general guidelines. If the crib mattress is at its lowest setting and your toddler's head and neck are above the rail when she is standing up, then she is tall enough to climb out of the crib and can no longer be safely left in the crib. Your baby is apparently large enough, old enough, and probably finds the crib too confining, especially if you find her standing up rattling her cage. You will find a variety of interesting baby beds at baby furniture stores. Expect frequent night waking for a while as she makes the transition from crib to bed. To minimize this, lie down with her in her new bed or next to her for a few nights as she gets used to it. Place one side of the bed against the wall and put lots of pillows on the other side or on the floor in case she rolls off. Detachable side rails that fit under the mattress may safely contain the sleeping child.

120. *Our nine-month-old baby wakes up to nurse several times a night. My friends advise me to let him cry it out, but I just can't do that. Should I let him cry?*

This is one of the most frequent questions we are asked. In order to answer this question in our book *The Fussy Baby*, we sent out questionnaires to several hundred parents. One of the questions was "How do you feel about the advice to let your baby cry it out?" Ninety-five percent of mothers responded that this advice did not feel right. From these results we concluded that this overwhelming proportion of mothers could not be wrong. The advice to let babies cry it out a little bit longer each night until they learn to fall asleep on their own has been in baby books since the early 1900s, and only recently have pediatricians begun to question its wisdom!

Remember, it is very easy for someone else to advise you to let your baby cry. They are not there at 3:00 A.M. They do not have any biological programming to respond to your baby as you do. Your baby's cry triggers an inner sensitivity which prompts you to give an immediate nurturing response and not to restrain yourself.

Letting your baby cry does two things: First, it causes your baby to feel that the cues that he has learned to trust and use to anticipate a response are no longer being responded to. This confuses him and may lessen his general trust of a responsive environment. Second, it does something undesirable to you. By restraining yourself from following your instincts, you desensitize yourself to your own biological intuition. In doing so you jeopardize one of the most valuable of all maternal qualities—sensitivity. When a mother says to us, as you did, "It bothers me to let my baby cry," we say, "Good, you are designed that way—you are a sensitive mother!"

We are not advising that letting a baby cry at night is always wrong, but that the decision must come from the parents. As you and your baby refine your communication network, you will develop a crying wisdom to know which cries need an immediate nurturant response and which cries can be left unattended for a few minutes, after which baby may resettle by himself. During the writing of this book our one-year-old, Stephen, began waking up several times a night to nurse. Martha was becoming exhausted. For three nights I comforted Stephen by walking and rocking him. Because he preferred Martha, he still cried, but he didn't cry alone! After three nights of "father nursing" he resettled more easily and awakened less. While parents occasionally report to us that letting the baby cry has worked, most parents report that it makes all of them a wreck. The baby gets angry, cries harder, and can't get back to sleep. Trust your sensitivity—it will never lead you astray. (See also question 121)

121. *Well-meaning friends and relatives have advised us that to get our baby to sleep through the night we should let her cry. They claim that she'll cry for an hour the first night, forty-five minutes the second, thirty minutes the third, and* *by the end of the week she will be crying less and sleeping through the night. We tried it once and we couldn't get beyond the first ten minutes. Both of us were rushing in to comfort a sobbing, shaking, and very scared baby. Boy, was she mad and did we feel guilty! We never tried it again, but why didn't it work and why did we feel that way?*

This restrained approach did not work because some rules of nighttime sensitivity were violated. Guilt is a healthy reaction when some inner parental instinct has not been followed. Although this approach does sometimes work, a lot depends upon the temperament of the baby and the sensitivity of the parents. Some babies easily adapt to developing alternative ways of soothing themselves back to sleep. Others have a definite set of expectations. They have a clear pattern of response in which they have learned to anticipate that distress will always be followed by comfort. They have learned that their cries will be listened to and they will be resettled by the person they have learned to trust. Their trust is so strong that their cries become equally strong until they receive their anticipated response. It sounds like you have this type of baby and that you are sensitive parents. A sensitive baby and sensitive parents are a good match of temperaments and promote a trusting personality development. Value the fact that your baby didn't give up and that you gave in. Also, don't feel that you have been manipulated by giving in. This is a question of trust, not who is manipulating whom. Continue to trust each other and you'll all continue to get along much better. (For sleeping inducing tips and alternatives to the cry-it-out approach see questions: 97, 98, 107, 111, 112, 116 and 120.)

122. *Our two-year-old wakes up like a bear. He seems angry and upset as soon as he gets out of bed in the morning. How can I help him start the day off on the right foot?*

You can help him start the next day off right by helping him end the previous day right—that is, by going to bed

peacefully. The last state of consciousness that a child is in
before drifting off to sleep is the state of mind that he will
most likely wake up in. This accounts for the old saying,
"He got out on the wrong side of the bed." If a child goes
to bed angry, is left to cry himself off to sleep, or is upset
when drifting off to sleep, he is likely to awaken with the
same attitude. Lie down with your child and sing lullabyes
or tell a caring, loving story and/or massage. Convey love
to your child before he drifts off to sleep. This may also
help influence the content of your child's dreams. The last
face your child sees before drifting off to sleep should be
that of someone he loves, and the last words he hears should
be "I love you."

123. *Our two-month-old is waking up a lot from her crib
in the other room. When I take her into our bed, she seems
to sleep better, but I'm afraid of creating a habit. I've heard
that once I start letting her into our bed, she'll never want
to leave. Is this right?*

Yes! When a child fits into any social situation in which she
feels right, she will not want to change that situation. For
example, if you like your job, you don't quit. If you have a
good marriage, you don't get a divorce. If your child feels
right—and it seems she does when sleeping with you—she
is not likely to want to go into her own bed for a year or
two. We advise you to enjoy your baby for the present and
don't worry about the future—your baby doesn't. As long
as you and your baby sleeps better and you all feel right
about it, this is the right decision for you. There is a time
for weaning for every baby. She will indeed leave your bed
when her time has come.

   To us this seems like your baby has a *need* to sleep
with you, not a habit. A need filled early will later disappear. Your baby will eventually wean from your bed when
she is able to comfortably sleep alone. Enjoy this closeness
while you can. She will be a baby for a very short time.

124. *Our new baby was waking up so often that the only way that both of us could get a good night's sleep was for me to take him into bed and let him sleep alongside me. That way when he woke up, I could get to him quickly and nurse him before both of us completely awakened. My husband is a very light sleeper, however, and the normal sounds of a baby being fed keep him awake. He exiled himself to the living room couch. He's not complaining, but our love life has suffered. What can we do?*

Part of becoming a new parent is learning to be sensitive to everyone's nighttime needs. The following is a letter we received from an experienced mother who worked hard to be both a good mother and insure a happy marriage: "The only way my baby and I could get any sleep was to sleep together. We nursed without either of us fully awakening. My husband, however, was too sensitive to the baby's noises and couldn't sleep with her in our bed. So he slept on the family room couch. We both had nighttime needs, too. Frequently when I was awake, I would go into the family room and join my husband for some special time together." We wonder what that husband must have felt the first night his wife greeted him with this nighttime surprise. It is so unusual for a new mother to initiate lovemaking that this mother's nighttime creativity surely helped her husband accept the family room couch. As a father of seven, I know that a realistic fact of having a new baby in the house is that fathers may expect to spend a few nights sleeping out of the bedroom until they get used to sleeping through normal baby noises. Until your husband gets used to your baby's nighttime noises, we suggest you surprise your husband as the mother did in this letter. (An alternative is the sidecar arrangement described in question 112.)

125. *My husband is afraid that allowing our baby into our bed might ruin our sex life. When should we worry about making love with our baby in our bed?*

The negative feelings about babies in bed during lovemaking are usually unwarranted. We don't believe that the love between parents adversely affects the product of their love. Embracing and showing affection between husband and wife is healthy in front of children at any age. Your main concern is about sexual relations while your baby is in your bed. Babies under six months have limited awareness of what is going on anyway, so lovemaking with your baby asleep in your bed is seldom a problem in the early months. In addition, many couples who have happily survived having their baby in their bed have discovered that the master bedroom is not the only place where lovemaking can occur. Every room in your house can become a potential love chamber. Another option is to carry your sleeping child into another room. A child who is in deep sleep does not awaken if gently moved to another bed in another room in the middle of the night. It is absolutely necessary that husband and wife find their private time together alone.

When children get older, we feel that they get two messages concerning the parents' bedroom: The door is open to them if they have a strong need to be with their parents, but there are private times when their mother and father need to be alone. You may employ the traditional "go watch cartoons" as you kindly but firmly request that your child leave your bedroom. Don't be afraid about hugging and kissing in front of your children. There is currently an epidemic of intimacy problems among teenagers and young adults. Counselors in sexuality problems feel that many of the sexual problems of today result from an inhibition of family members showing affection for one another.

126. *Our nine-month-old girl still has trouble sleeping through the night. She was a colicky baby for the first two months. I nursed her until I had to go back to work when she was four months, and now she is on formula. She cries out loudly and jackknives as she rolls on her side trying to*

*get off her tummy. She definitely seems to be in pain with
some type of gastric distress. How can I help her?*

The night waking pattern that you are describing seems to
indicate a milk allergy. The clue here is that your baby is
awakening in pain and not from being alone or emotionally
upset. The more we study night waking, the more we realize
that if you look hard enough you will find a physical cause
of painful night waking. Chances are high that your baby is
allergic to cow's milk formula, so the first thing we would
suggest is to change your baby to a soy formula. Around
thirty-five percent of babies who are allergic to cow's milk
are also allergic to soy. If this is the case, you may need to
use a nonallergenic formula such as Nutramigen or Preges-
tamil. Discuss this possibility with your doctor so that she
can suggest an alternative formula. If milk allergy seems a
possibility, try this simple test: Try a nonallergenic formula
suggested by your doctor for a period of two weeks. Meanwhile make a list of your baby's most worrisome symptoms.
If these symptoms disappear during the two-week trial
period, milk allergy is a possible cause. Then give your baby
the milk-base formula again. If the symptoms reappear, then
milk allergy is probably the cause. Also, breastfed infants
may exhibit these night-waking patterns if allergic to the
dairy products that their mothers drink.

127. *Our two-year-old boy still wakes up often. He was a
colicky baby and has never slept very well. He has been
restless at night and seems to be sometimes writhing as if
having a stomach ache. It has not grown any worse, but it
hasn't gotten any better either. He used to spit up a lot as a
tiny baby, but he doesn't do that anymore. I know something's bothering him at night, but I can't figure out what it
is.*

Apparently there is a physical reason for your child's night
waking. Milk or some other food allergy is a possibility (see
question 126). A recently discovered cause of night waking

which may apply to your child is the pediatric regurgitation syndrome, also called gastroesophageal reflex. In this condition your baby's esophagus (the tube going from the throat to the stomach) connects to the stomach at an abnormal angle. Therefore, when the stomach contracts, it pushes food and irritating stomach acids up into the esophagus instead of down into the intestines. The stomach acids irritate the esophagus, causing what adults call heartburn. In some cases we have recently had which were resistant to all other treatments for night waking, we have found that this syndrome was the cause. Medical tests are necessary to diagnose the problem, but the treatment is easy and the results are immediate. Reflex is treated by medications which relax the contractions of the stomach muscles and lessen the acidity of the gastric secretions. Discuss this possibility with your doctor if your child seems to have a physical reason for night waking.

128. *Our two-year-old wakes up frequently. Our older child was recently diagnosed as having worms. Could worms be the cause of our baby waking up. How do we find them?*

Yes, pinworms can cause night waking. To diagnose this, take a flashlight and exam your child's anal area at night. Spread the buttocks apart and look for the worms. Pinworms look like tiny pieces of white thread about a third of an inch long. The worms hatch after the pregnant female pinworm travels down the intestines and out the rectum to lay her eggs. The activity around the rectum which occurs at night results in intense itching, which causes the child to awaken and scratch the egg-infested area around her anus and buttocks. These eggs are picked up under the fingernails and transmitted to the child's mouth, to other children, and to other members of the household. The swallowed eggs then hatch in the intestines, mature, mate, and repeat the life cycle. Sometimes you won't see the worms, but you can see the scratch marks around your child's anus. If you can't see the worms but still suspect they are there, you can collect eggs in the following manner: Place a piece of tape sticky side out on a Popsicle stick and capture the eggs by pressing the sticky side of the tape against the anus at night. Take the tape to your doctor or a laboratory, where it can be examined under a microscope for pinworm eggs.

Treatment for worms is easy. A simple medication taken once by every member of the household and repeated again in ten days should completely eliminate the worms. In girls the pinworms can travel up into the vagina, cause vaginal irritation, itching, and scratching of the vaginal area, and can sometimes result in urinary tract infections.

129. *Our baby is nine months old and we haven't left him very often. Occasionally, however, my husband and I really want a night out alone. He has difficulty falling asleep with a baby-sitter, and when he awakens with a baby-sitter in the house, he is very upset and won't resettle. How can I solve the problem?*

Babies get very attached to the person who helps them drift off to sleep and who resettles them when they awaken. Some babies have stronger attachments than others, and these are least likely to accept alternatives. Here's how to help your baby sleep better with a baby-sitter in charge and help you better enjoy your night out: Get your baby familiar with a consistent baby-sitter. Let the baby-sitter watch how you resettle your baby. Instruct the baby-sitter that you want your baby put to sleep or resettled the same way. Remember, baby-sitters are substitute mothers. They may have to learn your mothering ways. If possible, try to get your baby to sleep before you go out. Leave a piece of your intimate apparel such as a bra or blouse next to your baby so that he has a familiar scent next to him when he wakes up. Leave a tape recording of yourself singing a song that your baby enjoys. Let the tape recording play continuously when you're away, or instruct the baby-sitter to turn on the tape when your baby begins to wake up. Be sure to leave your baby-sitter instructions not to let your baby cry it out.

You want your substitute caregiver to be sensitive to your baby too.

To get our infant to go to sleep for a baby-sitter we have successfully used the techniques of "pass the baby" and "wearing down." If your baby is used to being carried in a sling-type carrier (called baby wearing), shortly before the baby-sitter arrives, wear your baby around the house for a while. If he falls asleep in the carrier, put him down to sleep while still in the carrier (called wearing down—see question 131 for description) and then slip out. If the baby is quiet but not asleep, pass the baby—still nestled comfortably in the sling—to the sitter, who then wears the baby down to sleep. This smooth and familiar transition from one caregiver to another helps the baby more easily go to sleep for another person.

130. *Our two-month-old baby doesn't settle down well for anyone else but me. She won't go to sleep for anyone else and she cries whenever I leave her. My husband and I have not been out to dinner alone yet since our baby was born and I'm beginning to feel tied down.*

Your feelings are normal and shared by many new mothers. The key is to feel tied together and not tied down. There is nothing in the mother–baby contract that says you must stay at home. Home to a tiny baby is where you are. Take your baby with you. In the first few months you'll be surprised at how well babies settle down in restaurants. The difficulty will come later when your child is a toddler. Put your baby in a sling-type carrier and enjoy a good night out with your husband. Request a large booth in a quiet area of the restaurant. Try to time your outing around your baby's bedtime so that she can be nursed off to sleep discreetly in the carrier while in the restaurant, after which you can put her down on the seat of the booth. Sometimes taking along an infant seat and placing your baby asleep under the table is an alternative. A realistic fact of new family life is that previous dinners for two now become dinners for three.

With a bit of juggling, though, you and your husband can still go out to dinner while at the same time not anxious about how your baby is doing with the baby-sitter at home. We have consistently, through twenty-four years of marriage and seven children, managed to continue our custom of a weekly dinner for two, sometimes out, sometimes in.

131. *Our six-month-old is very difficult to get to sleep. I know he is tired, but he just doesn't want to give up. As soon as I put him into his crib he immediately wakes up. How can I get him to go to sleep more willingly?*

First-time parents may have been led to believe that the way a baby goes to sleep is that at some pre-assigned time you put the half-awake baby into the crib, pat her on the back, say "night-night," turn out the lights, and leave the room. The baby peacefully drifts off to sleep without much bother. This happens only in books and movies or for everybody else's baby, but seldom in real life. Most babies want or need to be nursed (meaning comforted) down to sleep in a care giver's arms. In our family we have used the custom of wearing down to put our reluctant sleepers to bed.

When you feel your baby is ready for bed—or you are ready to put him to bed—put him into a sling-type carrier and wear him around the house awhile. Use a wearing position which contains your baby the most, such as a deep cradle hold in which most of the sling covers him, shutting out almost all the stimulation from his environment. Wear your baby in the sling in the position that you have found to be the least stimulating and most sleep inducing. When he is in a state of deep sleep (recognized by a motionless face and limp limbs), lie down on your bed with baby still in the sling and gently slip yourself out of the sling. Allow the baby to remain in the sling, using it as a cover. Your baby may still seem to be restless while wearing down (this is called REM sleep, a lighter state of sleep in which he is more likely to awaken if you put him down and try to sneak out of the room). If this happens, keep your baby in the

carrier snuggled securely against your chest and lie down
with him on your chest while still in the sling. The rhythm
of your heartbeat and breathing motion will lull him into a
deep sleep, after which you can roll over and slip yourself
out of the sling. Your baby will usually stay asleep.

132. *Our two-year-old simply will not go to sleep. By nine
o'clock we are exhausted and she is still wound up. How
can we get her to wind down?*

Sleep is not a state you can force a child into. It must
naturally overtake the child. Here are some suggestions on
creating a sleep-inducing environment to help wind down
your wide-awake toddler: Begin the bedtime ritual earlier,
around seven o'clock. Avoid activities such as wrestling and
exciting play after this time. Try the following ritual: a
warm bath, a soothing story, and an oil massage while the
lights are dim and gradually getting dimmer. One parent
can be gradually dimming the lights as the other is winding
the toddler down. Use your bed or a large mattress on the
floor and lie down with your child, remaining there until she
is sound asleep. A tape recording of one of your child's
favorite stories or of yourself telling a story may sometimes
be used if you are not able to do the full ritual that night.
Here are some tips given to us by other tired but creative
parents:

1. If you have several young children who dislike going to
   bed, announce this game: "Whoever is in bed first picks
   the story."
2. Use an alarm clock or stove buzzer to signal "bedtime in
   five minutes."
3. The back rub game. "Plant a garden" on your child's
   back, using different touches for different foods which
   your child selects. Gradually lighten your stroke as you
   smooth out the garden.
4. Use an egg timer. "When all the sand hits the bottom,

the lights must go out." Your child may get tired watching the sand fall.

5. Bedtime stories. Choose books that strike your fancy too, books that you don't mind reading over and over again. Expect your child to cry, "Read it again." Choose books that emphasize sounds that are repetitive, rhyming, flowing, lulling, and comforting. As your child gets a little older she will enjoy your making up your own stories, but keep them monotonous. We use stories that are interesting in subject matter—i.e., fishing or baseball—but repetitive and involve counting: Billy caught one fish and pulled it in; then he caught two fish and pulled them in; etc. Usually by twenty fish (or base hits) one of you will be asleep.

6. Some children have trouble going to sleep because they are truly not tired. Providing an hour or two of outdoor exercise can give your toddler's body the physical exertion needed to build strong muscles, and it will also give her a reason to be tired and ready for restorative rest. Tension that is released through exercise cannot interfere with her ability to relax as bedtime approaches.

133. *Our three-year-old just doesn't want to go to bed until nine or ten o'clock. I know he is tired, and he is definitely cranky late in the evening. My husband, who gets home very tired from working late, feels I should be doing a better job of getting him to go to bed earlier. How can I accomplish this?*

There are three reasons why children don't want to go bed: fear of going to sleep, not wanting to be separated from you, and wanting time with the working parent at night. In this case it is the latter. Because of changing life-styles, rigid bedtimes are not as common or as realistic as they used to be. Decades ago, when most families lived in rural settings, the family got up early, worked together most of the day, and went to bed together early in the evening. Because today's parents are so busy and often do not have much time with their children during the day, children put their bid in for prime time with Mom and Dad at night, just at the time when the child is tired and the parents are too.

You might try the following: Give your child a nap late in the afternoon, so that by the time Dad arrives home both he and your child can enjoy some prime time together and you can get some much needed relief. Don't feel that you are breaking the rule if your child's bedtime is not until nine or ten o'clock or even as late as you go to bed. This unconventional bedtime may occur in particularly large and busy families or if the father does not get home until late. Babies often develop a sleep–wake schedule which helps them get the most time with their family. This is true in our own family with our youngest daughter, Erin. In the morning, our household is very busy with the other four children getting up and going off to school. Erin learned to sleep through this chaos and awaken around nine-thirty. The older children return home around three-thirty, so Erin learned to take her nap from three-thirty to five-thirty. The chaos settles down again around suppertime and Daddy's homecoming. By then Erin is awake and refreshed and ready to enjoy a full evening of prime time with her family. She then willingly falls asleep around ten or sometimes not until we go to bed.

The way a child goes to bed is more important than when he goes to bed. If you are a busy family and do not have much time with your child during the day, a later bedtime may be more realistic. If you do have a lot of time with your child during the day, a consistent and earlier bedtime is wisest. Studies have shown that children do better if they have a consistent bedtime rather than sometimes staying up late and other times being put to bed early.

134. *Our one-year-old baby wakes up frequently, and I am up and down all night long like a yoyo. We have tried everything and nothing works. The whole family is a wreck from not enough sleep. My doctor suggests a sleeping medication. Is this safe for babies?*

Yes. When used under the direction of a physician, sleep medications are safe and effective for inducing sleep in your baby. Parents and doctors are often reluctant to give sleeping medications to babies. Medications are a last resort. However, it seems as if you have a situation which may warrant the temporary use of such medications. If you have tried all the natural methods of getting your baby to sleep and nothing is working, it helps if you approach the situation by considering that you have a problem in which you don't like any of the solutions but must choose one. The use of sleeping medications, as suggested by your doctor, for one to three nights is appropriate. You should use caution when using sleeping medications for more than a few nights straight because they can become habit forming.

Sleep researchers find that most sleeping medications do not induce normal sleep. They interfere with the usual sleep stages and may leave a person tired the next day. In our experience the prescription medication chloral hydrate is the safest and most effective sleep-inducing medication for infants and children. Research has shown that this medication does not abnormally affect sleep stages. Other medications, such as antihistamines and barbiturates often have the opposite effect upon infants and children. They may wind them up at night instead of winding them down. Even the preferred sleeping medications such as chloral hydrate work in only about half the cases. Let's hope that your infant is in the half that responds. Be sure to use the amount and timing prescribed by your doctor. (For alternative methods of getting your baby to go to sleep and stay asleep. See questions 97, 99, 111, 112.)

135. *Our two-and-a-half-year-old likes to eat before going to bed. Which foods are likely to help her sleep better and which ones may keep her awake?*

Here are some tips for good bedtime snacks. Foods high in tryptophan (dairy products, fruits, turkey, and whole grains) are natural sleep inducers. A glass of warm milk, cheese and crackers, a bowl of cereal with fruit, naturally sweetened ice cream, and yogurt with fruit are good bedtime snacks. Sticky sugars (honey, caramel, syrup, raisins) should not be given to a child before bedtime because they promote dental cavities. With children who are sensitive to the effects of junk food, avoid foods that are high in cane sugar and artificial coloring. Cane sugar causes more ups and downs in the blood sugar, which may contribute to a disturbed night's sleep. The best kinds of sugars for children are the natural sugars in dairy products (unless a child is allergic to milk) and the fructose sugar in fruit. Caffeine-containing foods such as colas and chocolate may also interfere with sleep.

136. *My three-year-old wakes up often, and I feel it is because of my recent divorce. Could this be the case, and if so, what should I do about it?*

Yes, night waking is common following any prolonged separation from a parent either through death or divorce. Children often manifest disappointment by sleep disturbances. Expect your child's nap times to become more unpredictable and for her to prolong bedtime rituals. Expect your child to want to cling to you, mainly because of the fear that "Since Daddy is now gone, will Mommy leave too?" Your child may not want to go to bed alone or even nap alone, and you may often awaken in the morning and find your child asleep at the foot of your bed or even in your bed. Try the following: Picture nighttime from your child's viewpoint and realize that she needs extra security while she is going through this adjustment period. If she wants to sleep with you, let her. If she wants to prolong the bedtime ritual, accommodate her as much as you can. Tell your child reassuring stories at night about how much you love her and how you'll be right there when she wakes up in the morning. A child may need an extra bit of nighttime security for a night or two after she has spent a night or weekend with her father. It is very common for children not to sleep well when they are exposed to different sleeping arrangements and different life-styles in two homes. When your child sleeps in the non-custodial parent's home, send along familiar sleep-attachment objects such as a lambskin mat, a favorite blanket, or a teddy bear. Remember, children are more sensitive to family turmoil than they let on. And this disturbance is often manifested in unusual sleep habits.

137. *Our one-year-old sucks his thumb a lot before falling asleep. I'm worried that this may harm his teeth. How can I help him break this habit?*

Some children cannot drift off to sleep without the comfort of their thumbs. Others suck their thumbs habitually during most of the night. Most suffer no orthodontic problems from nighttime thumb sucking, but an occasional child puts enough pressure on his upper front teeth to cause an overbite. If you have a family history of orthodontic problems or either parent has an overbite, you may need to disrupt this nighttime habit. Here's how: Substitute this form of self-soothing with another. Lie down with your baby and nurse him to sleep if you are still breastfeeding, or sing to him and massage him to sleep. Watch how he sucks his thumb. If it is a very light sucking motion and he does not apply much pressure to his upper teeth, there is no need to worry. If he vigorously sucks his thumb and applies great pressure to his upper teeth, remove his thumb during sleep. You may need to lie down with him for an hour or two for a few nights, repeatedly remove the thumb, and substitute your own form of comforting.

138. *Our eight-month-old baby is hard to put to sleep, and sometimes I'm too exhausted to endure a long bedtime ritual. What about these talking devices that are advertised to put babies to sleep?*

In the past few years many ingenious devices have been invented to rescue parents from nighttime rituals. There are fuzzy teddy bears that have breathing sounds and sing lullabies. Personally we feel that whenever possible the care giver should put the child to sleep. We question the wisdom of habitually putting a baby to sleep to the sound of someone else's voice. The baby is a baby for a very short time and will need you to put her to sleep for only a tiny percentage of your life. We advise you to not spend money on these expensive sleep-inducing devices but rather give your baby yourself. You're much less expensive and much nicer!

139. *This is our first baby and I am confused about how tightly to wrap him at night. Should I swaddle him tightly or just use a loose blanket?*

Babies differ on how they like to be wrapped at night. Some babies like to "sleep tight" and like to be securely swaddled in cotton sheets or baby blankets. Other babies like to "sleep loose" and settle better in loose coverings which allow them more freedom of movement. Mothers have shared this swaddling tip with us: Cover your baby loosely during the day and swaddle him at night. This tighter nighttime swaddling may help condition him to associate swaddling with sleep, thus helping him settle better at night.

140. *Our six-month-old baby just will not wind down. I know she's tired—at least I'm very tired—but she refuses to give up. How can I get her to sleep?*

As we have frequently mentioned, sleep is not a state that you can force a baby into. The best you can do is create bedtime rituals that allow sleep to overtake your baby. Try the following:

1. A warm bath before bedtime and a soothing massage.
2. Swaddle your baby in her favorite blanket and use this blanket only for sleep.
3. Create a "moving bed." Many babies have difficulty making the transition from moving all day to the stillness of

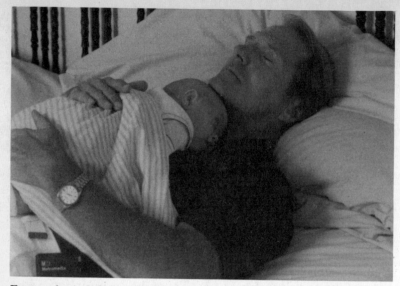

Even a fussy baby may settle easier when the father or mother "wears him down" to sleep.

sleep. Nursing and a rocking chair are usually a winning combination. If the back-and-forth motion of the rocking chair is not sufficient to lull your baby to sleep, then walk around with her for a while as you snuggle her across your chest or in a baby sling (see question 131).

4. Lie down with your baby and nurse her off to sleep. She may be ready to fall asleep, but doesn't want to go to sleep alone. After rocking and getting her almost asleep, lie down with her until she is in a state of deep sleep. You'll know that your baby is asleep when her sucking stops, her jaw loosens, and she lets go of the nipple so that you can easily ease it out of her mouth.

5. Some babies are sensitive to cold sheets. Warm the crib pad in the dryer or with a heating pad before putting your baby down on it.

6. If your baby is still small enough to fit in a cradle, the rocking may further lull her to sleep. When it comes to rocking, either in your arms or in a cradle, the rocking beat should be around sixty per minute. This is the heart-

beat rhythm that your baby has grown accustomed to in the womb. If she has outgrown a cradle, put rollers that don't squeak on your baby's crib and gently roll it back and forth around sixty times a minute. This technique is often used in hospitals, where all babies' beds have rollers.

7. Try the laying-on of hands. If your baby squirms and bobs her head up and down when you put her down to sleep, she is giving you the signal that she is not in a deep enough sleep to be left alone. Since her father has a bigger hand, he can lay his hand on the back of your baby's head or put one hand on her head and one hand on her back. The warmth of a secure hand may be the added touch that she needs to help her give up her silent protest and drift off to sleep. Patting your baby's back or bottom rhythmically at sixty beats per minute may add the finishing touches to the ritual of inducing sleep. Remember to remove your hands gradually, first one, then the other, easing the pressure slowly so as to not to startle your baby back to waking. Her sense of touch is probably keen. We have observed that when we put our hands on our babies, we must remove them very gradually. Let your hand hover just a bit over the baby's skin before removing it completely.

8. If all of the above fail, try freeway fathering. Put your baby in a safe car seat and go for a nonstop ride. When your baby has fallen asleep in the car, return home and place her in either her bedroom or yours, but don't try to remove her from the car seat or she will probably awaken. We have successfully used this technique many times. Recently our eighteen-year-old was baby-sitting our new baby while we visited their grandmother in the hospital. We came home and found that our teenager was out driving the baby around. A few minutes later, in came Jim holding the car seat full of a sleeping baby and proudly exclaiming, "I just tried freeway fathering. It worked!"

4

INFANT FEEDING AND NUTRITION

Feeding babies involves a knowledge of good nutrition, a knowledge of infant development, and creative "marketing." The answers in these chapters are geared toward these three goals. Over the past ten years infant-feeding practices have changed for the better. No longer do we feed babies according to the calendar, stuffing cereal into the reluctant six-week-old baby and feeling as though we have failed if our baby is not taking a full-course meal by six months. Today, infant feeding involves matching good nutrition with individual developmental readiness, which varies widely from baby to baby. Reading the feeding cues of your baby, introducing solid foods gradually, and encouraging self-feeding all lead to an important principle of baby feeding: creating a healthy feeding attitude. To a baby, eating is not only a nutritional necessity but a developmental and social skill. The more a baby enjoys the eating experience, the more efficiently he will advance in this skill. Eating is also a social interaction. A person is always at both ends of the feeding, whether it be by breast, bottle, or spoon. In this chapter we outline what foods to start with, when, and how much. We offer creative feeding techniques on how to get more food into your baby's tummy than on the floor. Quite honestly, early in our parenting career, mealtimes were our least favorite part of parenting. Once we taught our children the art of grazing—featuring our own Sears' nibble tray, an ice-cube tray filled with nutritious, colorful, bite-sized food varieties—we took the hassles out of mealtime. These and other feeding tips are sprinkled throughout this chapter. We will also clear up some popular misconceptions about feeding children fats and sugars— which ones are healthy, which are not. You will spend a lot of time feeding your baby during the first two years—enjoy it!

141. *Our four-month-old baby is breastfeeding and growing and gaining well. When should I start solid foods?*

During the first year you will spend more time feeding your baby than in any other parent–baby activity. Here are some suggestions to help you and your baby enjoy the first solid foods: Breast milk, a commercial formula, or a combination of the two contain all the essential nutrients your baby needs for the first four to six months. Parents sometimes get the urge to offer solid foods much earlier than the baby gets the urge to eat them. Pediatric nutritionists advise starting solid foods according to a baby's developmental readiness rather than her age. She may watch your food in transit from your plate to your mouth. She may reach for food from your plate. If your baby exhibits these signs of showing interest, here is a tip: Place a fingertip of mashed, very ripe banana on the tip of your baby's tongue. If her tongue goes in, accompanied by an approving smile, she is ready; if the banana comes right back at you, accompanied by a disapproving grimace, she probably is not.

Early on, babies have a tongue-thrusting reflex, meaning the tongue protrudes outward when any foreign substance is placed upon it. Between four and six months this tongue-thrust reflex diminishes and strained foods can be introduced. Around six months, babies begin to show two exciting developmental skills which makes feeding much easier: the ability to sit up in a high chair or on your lap and the ability to pick up small objects with fingers and thumb.

The upper end of baby's digestive tract (tongue and teeth) is not designed for early solids; nor are the rest of her insides. A baby's immature intestines are not equipped to handle a variety of food until around four to six months, when many digestive enzymes seem to click in. Pediatric allergists discourage early introduction of solids for the following reasons: The intestines are like filters, screening out the larger, potentially allergic proteins or digesting them into smaller, less allergic components. In the first few months a baby's immature intestines may allow potential allergens to seep into the bloodstream, thereby increasing the risk of the child developing more food allergies. Teeth seldom appear much before six months, so young infants' first solids should be pureed, strained, or finely mashed. As with so many aspects of parenting, observe your baby's feeding cues and not the clock. (See question 142.)

142. *Our five-month-old baby seems ready for solid foods, but I'm a bit anxious about what to give him and how much. Can you give me some guidelines?*

Start with solids which are closest to milk in taste and consistency. A very ripe mashed banana is a good starter food. Remember, your baby has to develop an entirely new feeding mechanism, from sucking-swallowing to tongue-mashing and swallowing. Start with a fingertip of mashed banana as a test dose. Place this small glob of banana on the tip of your baby's tongue, allowing him to get used to the new texture and taste. If you put the first solid foods too far back, your baby may be confused and have difficulty swallowing. Start with about one teaspoon of each new food, remembering that your initial goal is to introduce your baby to solids (new tastes, new textures, etc.), not to fill him up. Gradually vary the texture and amount to fit the eating skills and appetite of your baby. Some babies like solids of thinner consistency and want a larger amount. Some do better with thicker solids in smaller amounts. Baby foods are now available in a wide choice of textures and ingredients packaged in appropriate sizes for increasing appetites. Observe "stop signs" as well: Pursed lips, closed mouth, head turning away from the spoon coming toward him, are all signals that your baby does not want to eat right now. Don't force feed. You want him to develop a healthy attitude toward both the food and the feeding.

It helps if you develop a healthy attitude about infant feeding yourself. When beginning solids, think of infant feeding as helping your baby develop a new skill that you want him to enjoy. Don't be preoccupied with how much your baby takes. Offer solids at a time of day when he seems hungriest and/or you both need a change of pace. Mornings are usually the best time for offering solids to formula-fed babies, because you have the most time with your infant and usually do not have to worry about preparing a meal for the rest of the family. A breastfed baby should be offered solids when your milk supply is lowest, usually toward the end of the day. Since infants have no concept of breakfast, lunch, or dinner, when they receive what really makes no difference. The following are favorite starter foods for most babies: bananas, rice and barley cereal, applesauce, peaches, pears, carrots, squash, sweet potatoes, mashed potatoes, and avocados. We have written a booklet entitled "Baby's Garden—Nature's Guide to First Foods." To send for this free booklet, write to: Baby's Garden, 1251 E. Dyer Rd., Suite 200, Santa Ana, CA 92705.)

143. *Our five-month-old baby seems perfectly content with only breastfeeding. Our friends and my mother-in-law keep asking me, "What is she eating?" Must she have solids at this age or can I wait longer?*

If your baby is thriving well and shows no interest in solids, don't be in a hurry to introduce them. Although most babies do enjoy some solid foods by six months of age, some babies, especially breastfeeding ones, are content with only breast milk and don't need or want solids for a few more months. In our experience, breastfeeding mothers often start solids later than bottle-feeding mothers. Probably the reason for this difference is that bottle-feeding mothers are more time-oriented about infant feeding. If their babies take more formula more frequently, mothers often interpret this as a sign of needing solid foods, whereas breastfeeding mothers simply nurse more frequently to accommodate the baby. It sounds as if you have a baby who is content to receive all of her nutrition from your milk and delivered to her in the way she enjoys. After all, breast milk is simply specially processed solid foods, and your baby receives all her essential nutrients from your milk. Any developmental skill is best learned when it is initiated by the baby. The same goes for infant feeding. When your baby initiates signs of solid food readiness, that is the time to begin (See question 141.)

144. *Our six-month-old baby nurses from the breast frequently. It's been an easy and enjoyable method of feeding him. I'm really not looking forward to starting solid foods, but our pediatrician says it is time. Can you give me some tips on how I can enjoy feeding him solids just as I've enjoyed him breastfeeding?*

Breastfeeding is not only nutritional but also social and developmental interaction. Solid feeding can be as well. Consider solid food feeding as an addition to, not a substitute for, breastfeeding. Here's how both you and your baby can get the most out of this new relationship. Besides using your fingertip and a spoon to start solids, allow your baby to feed himself. Place a bit of mashed banana within grabbing distance on his table or high-chair tray. Make the most of your baby's rapidly developing hand skills. Around six months babies pounce upon anything of interest placed in front of them. You will notice your baby can soon pick up a morsel of food between his thumb and fingers and gradually bring it to his mouth. In the beginning stages of finding his mouth, the baby may have more misses than hits, resulting in much of the food being splattered all over his cheeks. Sharing the food with his face and shirt is part of feeding. Allow your baby the experience of trial and error; eventually practice makes perfect.

Allowing your baby to feed himself capitalizes on some new research on infant learning. A skill that is initiated by the baby has more learning value and attention-holding power than one initiated by the parent and simply participated in by the baby. Enjoy table talk. Talk to your baby during feeding. Talk about both the food and the procedure so that he learns to relate the words with the type of food and the interactions soon to follow. We have done this with our babies, frequently saying such things as "Matthew want carrots . . . open mouth!" as we gently approached his mouth with the solid-laden spoon. Talking to your baby during feeding also helps you know if he is truly interested in taking solids at a certain time. If his face lights up and his mouth opens as you talk, this gives you a clue that he is ready. Let the baby watch your mouth open; chances are he will mimic your facial gesture.

Reading the feeding cues of your baby, encouraging self-feeding, and advancing gradually all lead to an important principle of baby feeding: creating a healthy feeding attitude. To a baby, eating is not only a nutritional necessity but a developmental skill. The more a baby enjoys an experience, the more efficiently he advances in that skill. Infant feeding not only provides fun and nutrition for the baby; it also helps parents witness and enjoy their baby's rapidly developing hand skills. Feeding is a social interaction, not just a nutritional necessity. Enjoy it!

145. *We have a lot of allergies in our family. Because of this, I plan to breastfeed as long as possible. What precautions should I take when our son seems ready for solids?*

The longer you can wait to introduce potentially allergenic foods, the more developed your baby's intestines will be.

The more mature his intestines are, the better they filter out potential allergenic proteins or digest them into smaller, less allergenic substances. The least allergenic starter foods are: banana, rice and barley cereal, carrots, squash, sweet potatoes, and mashed potatoes. Citrus fruits and juices (oranges and grapefruit) should be avoided. Avoid mixed cereals and, for that matter, any packaged mixtures, because if your baby is allergic it will be more difficult to identify the allergen in mixed foods. Avoid egg yolk before nine months and egg white before one year. Delay dairy products and wheat as long as possible. In case your baby proves to be intolerant or allergic to a certain food, it is wise to space each new food about a week apart and keep a diary of which foods your baby may be allergic to. The usual signs of food allergy are: bloating and gassiness, a sandpaper-like rash on the face, runny nose and watery eyes, diarrhea and diaper rash, night waking, and generally cranky behavior.

146. *How much formula should our three-month-old be taking, and how often should I feed her?*

As a general guide, most infants need between two to two and a half ounces of formula per pound of body weight per day. Some days your baby may take more, some days less. If she weighs around thirteen pounds, then from twenty-six to thirty-two ounces is advisable. Most three-month-old babies require formula feeding about every three hours during the day and one bottle during the night. This amount also varies from infant to infant. Formula-feeding babies are easier to schedule than breastfeeding ones because infant formula is digested more slowly than breast milk, allowing the infant's tummy to remain full longer. A wise infant-feeding practice is to strive not to give your baby large volumes of formula in hopes of stretching out the feedings. Tiny babies have tiny tummies and are best fed with small, frequent feedings rather than with widely spaced, large-volume feedings.

147. *Our eight-month-old baby is still waking up at ten at night. I've heard that giving him plenty of solid food before he goes to bed may help him sleep through the night. Is this true?*

Generally no. Controlled studies in which babies of the same age were tested by giving one group solid foods before bedtime and the other group only formula or breastfeeding showed no difference in the amount of night waking. Despite these studies, some parents swear that it does help. If you have not been able to identify any other cause of night waking, perhaps some rice cereal and/or bananas may help your baby sleep a bit longer. As tired parents of seven, we too have considered this temptation but have not found it to work.

148. *Our two-month-old spits up a lot, but my doctor says not to worry. If she keeps on spitting up, when should I worry?*

Many babies spit up several times a day, and for most this is more of a nuisance than an indicator of an underlying medical problem. If your baby is gaining weight normally and seems generally well, if the spit-up is non-projectile (does not come out forcefully at a distance of one to two feet) and is not stained with yellow-green bile, you do not have to worry. Spitting up usually lessens around six to eight months, when babies spend most of their time in the upright position. Here are some warning signs that spitting up is more than a temporary nuisance and is becoming a medical problem: If your baby is obviously losing weight and showing signs of dehydration (needing fewer and fewer diaper changes each day), you should notify your doctor. If she seems to be in intense pain, showing projectile and bile-stained vomiting with every feeding, this is a medical emergency and you should seek medical attention immediately.

Here are some suggestions on lessening the nuisance

variety of spitting up: Feed your baby smaller but more frequent feedings. Burp her during the feeding (as you switch breasts, if you are breastfeeding), and keep her upright at least twenty to thirty minutes after each feeding.

If these measures don't help much, there is the possibility that the formula (or something in your breast milk) is not being tolerated. Ask your doctor to help you choose a formula that agrees more with your baby's stomach. If you are breastfeeding, consider what in *your* diet might be the culprit(s)—eliminate allergenic-type foods (dairy products and wheat top the list) for two to three weeks on a trial-and-error basis to see if you can pinpoint the offending food(s).

149. *Feeding our seven-month-old is a mess! The food is all over him, me, and the floor. How can I make feeding time a bit easier for both of us?*

Although a little mess is part of feeding (believe it or not, it has learning value), here are some tips on getting your baby to "clean up his act." If he tries to feed himself in the beginning stages, there may be more misses than hits, and much of the food gets splattered over his cheeks. Sharing the food with his face and shirt is part of the fun. Allow your baby to experience some trial and error. Expect him to treat solids as toys. He will watch the food splash on the floor and enjoy your reaction to this nutritious mess.

A variety of spoons and infant dishes (besides your fingers and the baby's hands) are available to help contain and guide the food. Here's a tip for getting most of the food where it belongs, a maneuver we call the "upper lip sweep." Place a spoon full of solids in the baby's mouth and allow his upper lip to sweep the food off as you gently lift upward and outward with the spoon. Getting your baby to open his mouth wider also helps keep more of the food in. Try the following: As you hold the spoonful of food in front of his open mouth, address your baby saying, "Baby (use name) want peas? Open mouth!" Open your own mouth in hopes that the baby will mimic your facial gestures. Talking about an interaction that is soon to follow is called a *setting event*; the words and gestures set up the familiar interaction that will follow. Setting events teach a baby to anticipate what will happen and allow him to communicate his desires. When he associates a spoonful of food with your open-mouth gestures, he will open his mouth a lot wider.

150. *Is it all right to let our nine-month-old feed himself his own bottle while lying in his crib?*

Generally no. This is a form of bottle propping, a procedure which we discourage for the following reasons: Babies should not lie down during bottle feeding, for the recumbent position may allow milk to enter the middle ear through the eustachian tube and cause ear infections. Leaving a baby unattended during a feeding is potentially dangerous if the baby chokes on the food and needs your help. Bottle propping also deprives both you and your baby of the valuable social interaction that occurs during feeding. Feeding is a social interaction, not just a nutritional exercise. There should be a person at both ends of the bottle.

151. *Our nine-month-old baby is breastfeeding and also likes solids. Should I feed her before or after breastfeeding?*

Experimental evidence from Sweden shows that solid food given with breast milk may interfere with the absorption of the iron from breast milk. In general, consider solid food as an addition to and not a substitute for breast milk. Offer solid foods at a time of day when your breast milk is lowest, usually toward the end of the day. Try offering solids between breastfeeding times rather than immediately before or after.

152. *How much juice should our nine-month-old baby drink?*

Babies usually like juice, but nutritionally they do not need large volumes of it. We discourage drinking a lot of fruit juice because it is a food with a low nutrient density, meaning it is high in calories for the amount of nutrition it contains. Undiluted fruit juice, for example, contains almost as many calories as the same volume of milk, but is much less nutritious. Juice is also less nutritious than the fruit itself because it lacks the beneficial fruit pulp. Because juice is less filling than milk, infants often consume a much larger quantity of juice without feeling full.

For a nine-month-old, apple juice is usually the favorite. Orange juice or grapefruit juice is usually too acidic. Vegetable juice is much more nutritious than fruit juice, but infants seldom like it. We recommend diluting apple juice with equal quantities of water, especially for the compulsive juice drinker. Avoid giving a baby a bottle of juice to go off to sleep. A combination of the sweet juice and rubber nipple can result in juice-bottle caries, dental cavities of baby's front teeth that result from the decay-producing sugar. For this reason, dentists recommend that juice not be given in a bottle but rather delayed until the baby can take juice from a cup—usually around a year.

153. *Is it all right to put cereal in our six-month-old's bottle?*

We do not recommend the feeding practice of adding solids to the bottle. Adding cereal to the baby's formula bottle usually requires significantly enlarging the nipple hole. The baby is taught to suck from the nipple, expecting a thin fluid substance to flow from the bottle. A sudden onslaught of a thicker substance may confuse her at a time when you are trying to teach her the difference between swallowing liquids and chewing and swallowing solids. We recommend giving solids on a fingertip or spoon so that the baby learns the correct tongue action of mouthing and swallowing the solid foods.

The main reason parents put cereal in a bottle is to "stuff" the baby, hoping to get her to sleep longer or to feed less frequently. We feel that stuffing a baby is an unwise feeding pattern.

154. *How old should our baby be before we can feed him regular homogenized cow's milk? Can we give him yogurt?*

The American Academy of Pediatrics recommends delaying non-formula cow's milk as a baby's primary beverage until after one year of age. Prepared formulas are much better suited to your infant's nutritional needs than cow's milk. Formulas are much closer to the composition of human milk and contain all the necessary vitamins. Most contain additional iron supplements that are so necessary at this age; cow's milk is very low in iron. Also, the younger the infant, the more likely he will be allergic to cow's milk. Formulas are more expensive than cow's milk, but by the time you add the cost of additional vitamins and iron, the cost of formula is only slightly more. Perhaps thinking of formulas as milk will lessen the urge to switch to cow's milk.

Yes. Yogurt gives all the nutritional benefits of milk, but with fewer problems. Yogurt is made by adding a bacterial culture to milk. This culture ferments the milk and breaks down the lactose into simple sugars which are more easily absorbed. This is important in infants who seem to be lactose intolerant. The milk proteins are also modified by the culturing process so that yogurt may be less allergenic than milk. Most infants enjoy yogurt around nine months.

155. *We have a history of obesity in our family and I don't want our baby to be fat. She is now one year old. Should I put her on a low-fat diet and use skim milk?*

No. A healthy diet for a one-year-old contains around 40 to 50 percent sugars, 30 to 40 percent fats, and 10 to 20 percent protein. Fats are a valuable energy source that babies need to grow. There are healthy and unhealthy fats. Healthy fats (also called monounsaturated fats) are found in fish, most vegetables and vegetable oils, and avocados. These foods provide essential fat nutrients for growing tissues. They contain either no cholesterol or good cholesterol—the type that does not clog arteries. Unhealthy fats, also called saturated fats, on the other hand, are those which do predispose heart problems by clogging arteries. Examples of unhealthy fats are greasy fats added to many packaged goods and fast foods, and animal fats such as those which marble and coat meat. Both the American Heart Association and American Academy of Pediatrics discourage low-fat diets in children under three. Even in babies and toddlers, concentrate on the healthy fats mentioned above. Unless recommended by your doctor, do not give skim milk to children under three years of age; use whole milk between one and two and low-fat milk between two and three.

Because of your family history, keep a check on your child's weight. This can be done by teaching her healthy eating habits. Avoid junk food. From one to two years of age your toddler will want to nibble often. Nibbling or grazing is a healthy eating habit, but let her nibble on nutritious snacks, not junk foods (see question 176). Be careful that your child does not use eating as a cure for boredom—a common cause of childhood obesity. Encourage physical activity if she has a sedentary temperament. Low-fat diets are occasionally prescribed in the child over two or three years of age if there is a strong family history of obesity, if the child herself is tending toward obesity, or if there is a strong family history of cardiovascular diseases from high blood lipids. In the latter case, have a blood-lipids profile performed on your child around three years of age. If there are abnormalities in your child's blood fats, your doctor can prescribe the necessary dietary adjustments.

156. *I think our nine-month-old drinks too much formula. Sometimes he drinks forty to fifty ounces a day and then seems to want more. He's not interested in solid foods and appears to be gaining a lot of weight. What can we do?*

Consider the use of a low-calorie formula. In the past several years formula manufacturers have introduced formulas which contain slightly less fat and fewer calories, much like the difference between whole milk and low-fat milk. Consult with your doctor about switching to a lower-calorie formula. Also, sometimes your child may be thirsty and not hungry. Offer him water or even some playful distractions when he cries for his bottle.

157. *Our one-year-old baby seems to get a lot of diarrhea whenever I give her cow's milk. Could she be allergic?*

Her problem could be a milk allergy, but probably it is a lactose intolerance. The primary sugar in cow's milk is lactose. Some infants do not have enough of the enzyme lactase in their intestine to digest cow's milk. (Breast milk contains this enzyme, cow's milk does not. This accounts for the feeling of bloating, gassiness, diarrhea, and a characteristic red rash on your baby's bottom. Strictly speaking, this is called a milk intolerance and not an allergy. Allergic signs to milk are more likely to be respiratory symptoms such as a runny nose, ear infections, and skin rashes. Many children do outgrow lactose intolerance and milk allergies.

158. *How much food should our nine-month-old be eating? Also, which is more important for him to have, formula or solid food?*

This varies a great deal from infant to infant. Some get their required nutrition mostly from formula at nine months; others lose interest in formula and eat a lot of solid food. It is much easier to insure proper nutrition with formula than with solid food. Try to give your infant balanced nutrition, meaning the proper amount of the basic nutrients. In general, a proper balance is 30–40 percent fats, 40–55 percent carbohydrates, and 7–15 percent protein. This balance is done for you in infant formulas, but if your infant is eating primarily solids and little formula at nine months, balanced nutrition becomes more difficult. In general, a nine-month-old infant takes between twenty-five and thirty-two ounces of formula per day, a volume which fills approximately half of his nutritional needs. By one year of age most infants receive at least fifty percent of their energy requirements from solids and the rest from formula or milk.

159. *Our six-month-old baby is formula fed. Should she also take vitamins?*

Look at the nutritional composition of the infant formula printed on the package, and you will notice that one can (32 oz.) of formula (either ready-to-feed or liquid concentrate) contains all the essential vitamins. If your infant averages one full can of formula each day, she probably does not need additional vitamins. If she does not consume at least one can of formula a day, additional vitamins are recommended. During the second year, if you switch to cow's milk or your infant takes less and less formula each day, vitamin supplements containing A, D, C, and also the B vitamins are recommended.

160. *I've heard that the iron in formula bothers some babies. Is it necessary to give our six-month-old iron-fortified formula?*

Controlled studies comparing iron-fortified formulas and formulas without iron have shown no difference in the degree of intestinal upset to infants. However, some mothers feel that additional iron does bother their babies. The American Academy of Pediatrics recommends that infants be given iron-fortified formulas during the first year. Unless your infant is bothered by the iron in the formula (constipation, diarrhea, abdominal pain), give your baby an iron-fortified formula. The iron in infant formulas often gives a baby's stools a greenish color. This color is of no significance. During the second half of the first year iron-rich foods (iron-fortified cereals and meat) can be used as other sources of iron in your infant's diet. Iron is necessary to make hemoglobin in your baby's blood. If he doesn't get enough iron, his hemoglobin will be low, a condition called anemia. This may cause him to be tired, pale, not grow well, and be more susceptible to infections.

161. *Should our one-month-old, formula-fed infant be getting fluoride supplements?*

If you are using ready-to-feed infant formula, a fluoride supplement is necessary. If you mix the formula with your tap water, check with your dentist about the fluoride content of the drinking water in your community. In areas where the fluoride content of drinking water is less than 0.3 parts per million, fluoride supplements are necessary. The American Academy of Pediatrics recommends that fluoride supplements be given to babies beginning at birth and continuing until ten to twelve years of age in areas where the fluoride content of the drinking water is low. Fluoride supplementation has been found to lower the incidence of tooth decay in children. Be sure that you strictly adhere to the dosage of fluoride prescribed by your doctor, since an excessive dose of fluoride can actually harm your child's teeth. Even though you do not yet see teeth in your one-month-old, the enamel is forming on the teeth inside the gum, so fluoride supplementation should begin at birth. At this writing, fluoride supplements are still recommended according to the above guidelines. Since new information in the future may be contrary to this recommendation, we advise checking with your doctor about fluoride.

Whether breastfeeding babies should receive additional fluoride is still under study. Some studies show that the frequency of dental caries in breastfed infants who are not supplemented with fluoride is identical to that of infants who are formula fed *and* supplemented with fluoride. However, fluoride taken by the mother does not pass in sufficient quantities into the breast milk. It is noteworthy that there have been some cases of fluorosis (damage to the enamel) in the teeth of breastfeeding infants who were given the usual dosage of fluoride supplements from birth on. Until this question is settled, the Committee on Nutrition of the American Academy of Pediatrics recommends that fluoride supplements be given to the breastfeeding infant beginning at six months of age, rather than at birth.

162. *Is it safe to give our baby megavitamins?*

Consider vitamins a medicine. You would not consider giving your baby any more medicine than your doctor prescribed. Any medicine must pass two tests: It must be safe and it must be effective. Parents usually ask about the use of megavitamins containing Vitamin C. Neither the effectiveness nor the safety of high doses of Vitamin C has been proven. We definitely do not recommend giving megavitamins to infants or children. Excessive doses of some vitamins, such as A, D, and E, can actually make your infant sick. Always follow the dosage of vitamins on the package or as your doctor prescribes.

Multivitamins (Vitamins A, B, C, and D) used in the dosage prescribed by your doctor, are safe. Formulas contain enough vitamin supplements (see question 159), and breastfeeding infants seldom need vitamin supplements. Your doctor may prescribe vitamin supplements if your baby's diet or eating habits seem to warrant additional nutrition. Some nutritionists advise additional vitamin D during sunless winter months.

163. *At our one-year-old's checkup, the doctor said his blood count was a bit low and put him on iron drops. What foods should I be giving him that are high in iron?*

Iron-rich foods in order of iron content are: liver, fish, beef, poultry, prunes and raisins, iron-fortified cereals, red beans, green leafy vegetables, and egg yolk. In general, the iron in meat, poultry, and fish is better absorbed than that in vegetables or egg yolk. While the latter is high in iron, this iron is bound to the egg yolk, meaning that much of it is not absorbed through the infant's intestines. Giving Vitamin C-rich foods, such as Vitamin C-enriched infant juices, along with the meal or snack containing iron-rich foods enhances the absorption of iron from these foods.

164. *We are both vegetarians and in good health. Is it all right for our eighteen-month-old baby to be on a vegetarian diet?*

The major problem with vegetarian diets in children is that vegetables are low in iron, thus leading to iron-deficiency anemia or "low blood." Though green leafy vegetables and beans are sources of iron, the iron in vegetables is not well absorbed by the human intestines. If you do not wish to give your child red meat, fish is very high in iron and an excellent alternative to meat. If you insist upon giving your child a vegetarian diet, consider the following: Giving Vitamin C-enriched juices along with vegetables may enhance the absorption of iron. Encourage high-iron, no-meat foods such as prunes, raisins, green leafy vegetables, and red beans. Ask your doctor to check your baby's hemoglobin (the amount of red blood cells, which determines whether or not she has enough iron in her blood) approximately every three to six months between ages one and three. If her hemoglobin is in the low or low-normal range, your doctor may prescribe iron drops.

165. *Our one-year-old is a compulsive milk drinker. He would drink two quarts of milk a day if I let him. He is only slightly overweight, but should I be worrying?*

There are two concerns with compulsive milk drinkers: too many calories and too little iron. Since milk is low in iron, a child who is a compulsive milk drinker runs the risk of iron-deficiency anemia. Although dairy products are generally a stable source of nutrition for a growing child, they are low in iron. If your child is also eating iron-rich foods (e.g., meat and fish) and your doctor checks his hemoglobin and finds it to be normal, you need not worry. Concerning the calorie question: Consider switching from whole milk to low-fat milk, which has much fewer calories. During the second year many compulsive milk drinkers switch from being drinkers to eaters once they learn the fun they can have with finger foods.

166. *Our two-year-old just won't drink her milk. Where will she get the calcium that she needs?*

It is interesting that some children who refuse to drink milk are actually allergic to milk. They refuse milk because it gives them intestinal discomfort. Calcium deficiency is rare in North America because some calcium exists in almost all foods. A toddler requires approximately 800 milligrams of calcium a day. Alternative sources of calcium include: canned salmon, pinto beans, tofu, broccoli, sardines, kale, soybeans, avocados, blackstrap molasses, legumes, green leafy vegetables, pasta, grains, and fruits. If your baby eats these calcium-containing foods and seems to be growing well, calcium supplements should be unnecessary. If she refuses these foods, consider a calcium supplement. Check with your doctor regarding vitamin supplements.

167. *I hear so much about sugar being bad for a child. Do I really have to keep my two-year-old son away from sugar?*

No! Sugars (also called carbohydrates and starches) are a necessary energy source for the growing child. Around fifty percent of child's diet should be in the form of healthy sugar. Healthy sugars are those contained in fruit, vegetables, grains, and dairy products. Unhealthy sugars are composed of the table sugar contained in icings and candy, for example. Some children are vulnerable to behavior effects of overdoses of unhealthy sugars, the so-called "sugar blues." These unhealthy sugars enter the bloodstream rapidly, giving the child a high blood-sugar level. This triggers the insulin cycle, which rapidly uses up these sugars and results in a rapid fall or low blood-sugar level. A child's moods often parallel the blood-sugar level, giving them highs and lows. This is why you may notice that your child's behavior deteriorates just before the next meal is due, because his blood sugar is low. Healthy sugars, such as fructose contained in fruits and vegetables, enter the bloodstream more slowly, do not trigger the insulin cycle the same way unhealthy sugars do, and do not leave the bloodstream so rapidly. In other words, the more healthy sugars provide a more steady supply of fuel rather than the highs and lows of unhealthy sugars. Less healthy or unhealthy sugars are also known as empty calories, meaning that sugars like icings and frostings contain only sugar and not other nutrients found in healthier sugars such as fruits.

Babies are born with a sweet tooth. One of the sweetest baby foods is breast milk. If you feed your child primarily healthy sugars during the first few years he gets used to feeling right when eating right and feeling wrong when eating wrong. If a sugar behaves badly inside the body, the child often misbehaves on the outside. Parents, you're the taste makers for your children. If you bring up your child on healthy sugars during the early years, when he gets to that inevitable first birthday party around three years of age and out comes the frosting-covered birthday cake with all the unhealthy sugared flowers on it, he may take one piece but refuse a second. Children who have been used to a steady diet of healthy sugars do not like the uncomfortable feeling they get from an overdose of unhealthy sugars. These children will get candy, chocolate, and icing as part of normal living, but the difference is that they will not overdose on it.

168. *What foods may not be safe for our two-year-old?*

The most common foods which may cause choking are the following:

- nuts
- popcorn kernels
- hot dogs
- raw carrots
- large seeds
- coffee beans or any other hard bean
- hard candy

Sometimes a young child may choke on stringy or coarse meats. Cut meats into very small pieces and mash coarse meats. Discourage the child from stuffing her mouth too full and laughing or crying with a mouthful.

169. *Our two-year-old gets black stains on his teeth. Could this be from vitamins?*

Vitamins that are high in iron or iron drops may cause a temporary dark stain on your toddler's teeth. This stain can be minimized by administering the drops farther back on his tongue, rinsing his mouth with water afterward, and brushing frequently. Iron causes a temporary green stain on the teeth just as it causes green stools. Both are of little significance.

170. *When should I introduce cup feeding to our baby?*

We like your term "introduce," which implies making any change smoothly and gradually. Going from bottle to cup requires a completely different mouthing orientation and better coordination in swallowing. Most babies take juice or milk from a cup between eight and twelve months. Begin with a trainer cup, which is almost spill proof and has an easily mouthed spout. The baby can hold this cup with both hands and sip a little at a time. Spout cups allow an easier transition from bottle to cup, since the amount of fluid baby gets does not overwhelm her. If she sputters a lot while drinking from a cup or makes a continual mess, then she is not yet ready to use a cup. In general, make feeding easy

and enjoyable for both you and your baby, and introduce
any new form of feeding according to your baby's development and not the calendar or the clock.

171. *I've heard that breastfeeding for a long time lowers
my child's risk of orthodontic problems. Is this true?*

Yes. Some orthodontists have told us that they can tell
whether a baby has been bottle or breastfed, and for how
long. Breastfeeding contributes to proper jaw alignment
because of the different pressures exerted on the jawbones
during sucking. Breastfed infants have fewer cavities because
of the nature of the milk and the natural rinsing action that
occurs during breastfeeding. A baby is required to use many
more oral facial muscles during breastfeeding than during
bottle feeding. A breastfeeding baby is less likely to develop
tongue thrusting (habitually pushing the tongue outward
against the upper teeth) because a breastfeeding baby must
learn to position his tongue properly during feeding,
whereas a bottle-feeding baby does not have to be so exact
about proper tongue placement. Nighttime breastfeeding is
becoming more widespread in Western cultures. If your
baby night nurses, brush his teeth the next morning. While
not nearly as common as night bottle cavities (see question
161), nighttime breastfeeders do get cavities. (For more
advantages to breastfeeding see question 45.)

172. *Our six-month-old looks very chubby. She is solely
breastfed and I'm not worried, but my friends are making
comments about her weight. Should I worry?*

Some babies, both breast- and bottle-fed, appear very chubby
during the first year. Providing their nutrition is appropriate, many of these babies begin losing this chubby
appearance between six and eighteen months, when they
begin crawling and walking and normally eating much less.
In wondering whether or not to worry about your chubby

baby becoming a fat child, consider whether or not she has the following risk factors:

1. The body type of the parents is the highest determinant of the risk of obesity. If both parents have an ectomorph (tall and lean) body type, it is unlikely that your infant will become fat. If one or both parents have an endomorphic (short and wide) body build, this increases the risk of the child becoming obese. Mesomorphs are somewhere in between.

2. Is your family tree littered with obesity? If the predominant body type of your family tends toward the ectomorph, obesity is less likely than it is with an endomorph family history.

3. Since your baby is totally breastfed for the first six months, this chubbiness should gradually subside over the next six months. Around six months the fat content of breast milk begins to automatically diminish as if there is a natural safeguard against breastfed babies becoming too fat. (See also questions 76, 81.)

173. *My friend's nine-month-old baby has anemia. My baby is about the same age. What is anemia and how can I prevent my baby from getting it?*

Anemia means low blood, specifically low hemoglobin in a baby's red blood cells. The most common cause of anemia in infants is an iron-deficient diet. Red blood cells need adequate supplies of iron in order to make hemoglobin. If your baby does not have enough iron in his diet he will become anemic. Iron deficiency may cause him to be tired, pale, not grow well, and be more susceptible to infections.

The good news is that the rate of anemia in children in the U.S. is dropping. The Journal of the American Medical Association recently published a study of nearly a half million children ages six months to five years, enrolled in WIC (Women, Infants and Children) programs. This study showed that the rate of anemia has dropped by almost two thirds from 1975 to 1985. Researchers cited trends toward more breastfeeding as a factor. Breastfeeding is beneficial because fifty percent of the iron in breast milk is absorbed by the infant. In contrast, the infant may absorb only four percent of the iron in iron-fortified formula. The most common age for iron-deficiency anemia to appear is nine to eighteen months. The following are ways that you can prevent this type of anemia from developing in your baby:

1. If you are formula feeding, use an iron-fortified formula for at least one year. Because cow's milk is low in iron, the American Academy of Pediatrics advises avoiding cow's milk as a beverage in infants under one year. If you are breastfeeding and plan to wean under a year, wean your baby to an iron-fortified formula instead of cow's milk.
2. Ask your doctor to check your baby's hemoglobin around nine months. This is usually routinely done at your baby's nine-month checkup.
3. Give your baby iron-rich foods (see question 164 for a list of these foods).

174. *We enjoy eating out, but our eighteen-month-old is a real nuisance at restaurants. Any suggestions on keeping him quiet?*

We also enjoy eating out and have been through the restaurant routine with our seven children. In fact, at this writing, we frequently take our eighteen-month-old to restaurants. First of all, choose a time to eat when the baby's behavior is usually at its best, or sleepiest. If you know that you are going out that evening, either push back his afternoon nap so he may fall asleep in the restaurant or push forward his nap so that he takes a long nap just before you are ready to go out. Taking a baby out to eat during what parents humorously call "happy hour"—5:00 to 7:00 P.M., when most babies show their worst behavior—is usually doomed to failure.

Feed your baby before you go out. Taking a hungry

baby into a restaurant is also asking for trouble. When your
child gets a little older, the term fast food will take on new
meaning. You will want to take your baby to a restaurant
that serves food quickly. If you choose a restaurant with a
more leisurely pace, order your baby's food right away to
be served before yours arrives, or take along some of his
favorite nibbles to munch on while waiting for your dinner.
Order or take along food that he cannot make a mess with.
Choose a restaurant where babies are socially acceptable—
a family-type restaurant which, admittedly, is usually noisy
enough that other families do not mind the happy noises of
children. Remember, a bored child is usually a nuisance in
a restaurant. Take along some of his favorite toys. Babies
love to bang utensils, an annoying sound in restaurants.
Take along his own plastic utensils. We notice that more
and more families are taking babies along with them for
many social occasions, resulting in parents learning creative
ways to make babies socially acceptable and in babies catching the spirit and becoming more enjoyable to be around.

175. *We travel a lot and our two-year-old has a ravenous
appetite. She's always eating. Any tips on infant feeding
and traveling?*

Feeding the hungry junior traveler requires a combination
of balanced nutrition and creative packing. Our diaper bag,
even on short shopping trips, often looks more like a lunch
box than a diaper container. Take along fresh fruit that can
instantly be peeled and served. The most nutritious ready-
to-eat fruit is an avocado. At a recent parenting conference
you could pick out the parents from California—they had
avocados in their diaper bags. Cut the avocado in half and
you have an "avocado boat." You can scoop it with a spoon
or finger feed it, mash it, spread it on bread or crackers,
even let your child dip other vegetables into a mashed avocado dip. Bananas are another ideal diaper bag food for
traveling. If your child is a grazer, several tiny plastic bags
filled with O-cereals will keep her busy and satisfy her hun-

ger. Baggies of cereal are also a great attention-holding food during long trips.

176. *Our eighteen-month-old is an extremely picky eater. How can I get more food into him?*

This is one of the most common complaints of feeding a toddler. A knowledge of some basic principles of toddler nutrition and usual eating habits will help. During the first year babies eat a lot because they grow a lot; you are used to him eating quite a bit. Whereas the average infant triples his birth weight by one year, the normal toddler may increase his weight by only one third or less between his first and second birthday. The toddler also begins to show a proportionately greater increase in height than in weight as he uses some of his excess baby fat for energy. This normal slimming down that occurs during this time may further increase parents' worry that their child is not getting enough to eat. In essence, a toddler's eating patterns change as his growth patterns change.

Changes in motor and emotional development also lead to changes in eating patterns. Three meals a day is an adult pattern. Toddlers are too busy to interrupt their relentless exploration to sit for long. Small, frequent feedings are thus more compatible with his schedule, and many nutrition experts think it may be the healthiest way to eat anyway. In another respect, the term *picky eater* is well deserved. The thumb and forefinger pickup, a fine motor skill which develops toward the end of the first year, also influences toddler eating patterns. The toddler delights in practicing this important new skill by manipulating foods, picking up small bits of edible items from a plate or high-chair tray.

The do-it-myself attitude so characteristic of toddler independence influences feeding patterns too! Your toddler may no longer let you feed him, but will probably prefer to feed himself. Accept the inevitable dawdling, spilling, and messing as part of the feeding game. Since toddlers also love to imitate adult eating patterns, capitalize on these desires by buying your child his own little dish, spill-proof cup, and utensils. Set his dinnerware on his high chair. When he sees everyone sitting at the table eating, he will most likely want to join you with his own tools and at his own pace.

Toddlers need between eight hundred and one thousand calories per day from one to two years of age, but they may not eat this exact amount every day. Your toddler may eat well one day and eat practically nothing the next. He may like fresh vegetables one day and refuse them the next. This patternless eating is normal, but if you average his food intake over a week or month, you may be surprised that his diet is more balanced than you thought. Remembering that feeding your baby from one to two years requires a combination of good nutrition and creative marketing, the following suggestions will help your toddler thrive:

1. Make "grazing" easy. Nibbling and snacking throughout the day is sometimes the best way to insure proper nutrition. In our home, we have achieved some success in feeding our toddlers by displaying an ice-cube tray or muffin tin, called a nibble tray, with various bits of colorful, nutritious food groups (marketed as a "rainbow lunch") and labeled with playful names a two-year-old understands: cheese blocks, avocado boats, banana wheels, carrot sticks, whole-wheat bread sticks, apple slices with peanut butter, etc. The behavior of toddlers and young children often parallels their eating patterns. Parents often notice that a toddler's behavior deteriorates toward the end of the morning or mid afternoon, that is, between meals. Snacking minimizes blood-sugar swings and lessens the resulting undesirable behavior.

2. Finger food and dips are favorites. Make a nutritious dip consisting of a base of mashed cottage cheese, yogurt, whipped fruit and vegetables, avocado dip, or even a nutritious salad dressing. Your toddler is more likely to eat his chunks of vegetables if he is able to dunk them into his favorite sauce.

3. Make foods easy to eat. In addition to the above mentioned dipping and nibble tray, respect the fact that small children have small tummies and less well-developed chewing and swallowing skills than we have. Cut the foods into bite-size pieces. Make pâté out of meat that is hard to eat and spread it on a favorite cracker.

4. Encourage foods with high nutrient density (a lot of nutrition per unit calorie): vegetables, avocados, legumes, meat, poultry, fish, and grains. Fruits have a lower nutrient density and juice has even less. If your toddler prefers to "drink his meal," try making "smoothies" of yogurt blended with fresh fruit.

Your goal as parents is to be in charge of what your toddler eats and to make nutritious foods available to him in a variety of ways. You should not take responsibility for how much your child eats. Remember that toddler feeding, like language development, is not a task to be forcibly learned but a skill to be enjoyed.

5

FATHERING

$\mathbf{O}$ver the past decade a father's role in child care has changed—for the better. As more mothers are sharing income earning, more fathers are sharing child care. Most men, however, are not prepared for this new role. The answers in this chapter will help dads become more involved in the care of their children. A popular fathering myth we wish to get rid of is the erroneous assumption that fathers are just substitute mothers. Men are not better or worse at nurturing than women; they nurture differently and their babies profit from this difference. In this chapter I (Bill) share with you some uniquely male nurturing tips which I have learned in fathering our seven children and some time-tested baby-comforting tips that other fathers have shared with us.

In the you-can-have-it-all commercial world, fathers are torn between professional success and family success. Dads, let me share a realistic fact of fathering life with you, which, pitifully, took me six children to discover—you can't have it all. Women can't; neither can men. Some juggling between work and home is necessary. Fathers feel the economic

154

pressure to put bread on the table, yet often do not have time to be present at the table. In this chapter you will find some career-juggling tips. A simple theme of many of the answers is the point that fathers, by their unique way of nurturing, play an important role both in the growth and development of their babies and as a role model for their older children. Having thrived and survived twenty-three years of fatherhood, I know the good things that babies do for fathers. Nothing matures a man like fathering a bunch of kids.

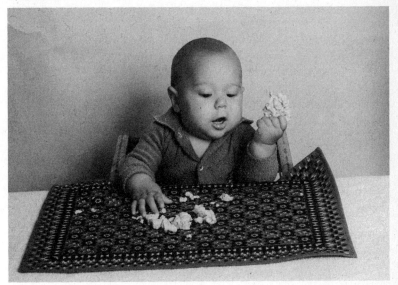

Babies can practice new motor skills while snacking on finger foods.

177. *I'm attending childbirth classes with my wife and am preparing to be what is called a labor coach. I am uncomfortable with this role; is it really necessary?*

I feel that men may coach sports but not laboring women. Expecting fathers to take on the role of labor coach may be asking more than they are ready to handle. After all, a man is not biologically equipped to understand the process of birth the way another woman who has herself experienced childbirth can. Do what you do best: Provide love and moral support. Hire someone else as a labor coach, a woman who has had some training or experience in midwifery or childbirth education. The following is a letter we received from a father who faced this coaching dilemma: "When my wife went into labor I wanted to share in our baby's birth. I wanted to experience, as much as I could, as a male, the joy of giving birth. We had attended childbirth classes and learned a lot of technical maneuvers. But when the time came, I forgot most of what I had learned and decided to act on my feelings by simply comforting and loving her through labor. Whenever my wife showed that a contraction was coming on, I would embrace her as gently as I could. I held one arm around her and placed my other hand on 'the bulge,' as I had affectionately termed this little person inside. As she labored I felt her arm squeeze me tightly and sometimes her fingers dug into my back. The more she dug in, the harder I could feel her uterine muscles contract. She felt better having me there and I felt I was playing a part in helping her labor progress."

178. *I have not been particularly close to my father over the years, and I don't want this to happen to our baby. We are expecting our first child in a few months, and I've heard that fathers can begin getting close to their baby by talking to their baby before birth. How does this work?*

Talking to a baby in the womb is an exciting area of research. The jury is still out as to how much the prenatal baby truly hears. Scientists claim that she can hear voices by at least the sixth month of pregnancy. Some researchers even feel that the pre-born baby hears her father's voice better than her mother's. The reason for this may be because the low-pitched, resonant male voice transmits better through the fluid-filled medium in the womb. Talking to your prenatal baby is a lot of fun. Let yourself go, saying whatever comes into your mind, such as: "Hi, baby, this is

Daddy. Can't wait to meet you!" Studies have shown that babies whose fathers talk to them before birth attended better to their fathers' voices during the newborn period. Get used to talking to your baby before birth and you'll have a lot more fun doing so after birth.

179. *I really want to be involved in the birth of our baby and am attending childbirth classes with my wife. How else can I help her?*

Your vital role in childbirth is to insure, as much as you are able, that your wife has the opportunity to follow the natural signals of her body during childbirth. Attending natural childbirth classes helps her tune in to her body's signals. Often the schedules and routines of hospitals' labor and delivery units do not encourage mothers to truly follow their bodies' signals, so this is where you can play an important role: Encourage your wife to move around during labor. Help her assume the laboring position in which she feels the most comfortable. Help her try standing, sitting, walking the halls, leaning over a table, getting on all fours, even squatting. Lying on her back during most of labor is not only the most uncomfortable position for a mother, but may also slow the progress of labor. Be tuned in to your wife's needs. Be ready with pillows when she needs them for support. Rub her back. (A four-inch paint roller is excellent for back massage.)

Spare your wife the hassles. A laboring woman is not always rational and diplomatic with the attending medical personnel. She shouldn't have to be. Her focus should be on her own needs and her body's signals. Any hassles with the attending personnel (paperwork, routines, hospital policies) should be taken care of by you. Remember, too, a laboring mother is particularly vulnerable to suggestions that she may not be making progress as fast as expected ("Tsk, tsk, still only six centimeters dilated"). If you sense a negative dialogue developing between your wife and the attending personnel, step in and redirect the communication in a more positive direction.

180. *I love my wife and new baby dearly, but I still feel left out. All my wife does is nurse and hold our baby. She doesn't seem interested in anything else, and we haven't made love for weeks. I'm beginning to feel there's something wrong with me. Do all first-time fathers feel this way?*

Your feelings and those of your wife are both common and normal. Perhaps an explanation of the biological reasons why new mothers behave the way they do may help you understand your wife's apparent preoccupation with your baby. A woman is endowed with two sets of hormones, sexual and maternal. Prior to birth and even sometimes prior to pregnancy, your wife's sexual hormones were at higher levels than her maternal hormones. After birth the reverse is true. Although this basic biological arrangement may not be convenient for you, it is nevertheless designed for the good of your baby. You may further understand your wife's behavior if you consider how you would have designed the perfect mother–infant care system. Since I have survived my wife's hormonal changes through seven babies, I have developed a theory as to why these changes occur. And during my years as a pediatrician and as a father, I have learned that babies do what they do because they are designed that way and mothers do what they do because they are designed that way. Your wife's shift of attachment from you to your baby is part of the normal design that insures that your baby will be well mothered to his fullest potential. One day I was explaining this to a left-out new father who commented, "This seems to be part of the for-better-or-for-worse clause in the marriage vow: Better for baby, worse for daddy." Fortunately, that's an over-simplification. Just because your wife seems disinterested in sex, don't feel that this means that she is disinterested in you. In addition to the hormonal reasons for her apparent sexual disinterest, another reason is probably that she is simply tired. Mothers we have interviewed have described an end-of-the-day feeling as being "all touched out," or "all used up" by the incessant demands of the new baby. This does not mean that you are being replaced by your baby but that some of the energies previously directed toward you are now being redirected. During the first few months after birth (and sometimes until after weaning) many wives do not have the energy to engage in a high level of intimacy both as a sexual partner and as a mother. Be patient, though, these energies will eventually be directed back toward you. Here are some tips on how you can help: I call the first few months after birth the season of the marriage, a season to parent. Become a supportive, sensitive husband during these early months when your wife is going through the many adjustments of motherhood. Help her with the many household chores or hire domestic help. Give her many "I understand" and "I care" messages. Meanwhile you are building up your wife's sexual interest in you. If you tend to this season of the marriage with care, you will later reap the harvest of a much richer sexual life and a more mature marriage. (See question 181.)

181. *It's been three months since the birth of our baby, and my wife still isn't interested in sex. Sometimes I feel that she's not even interested in* me. *What can I do?*

Much of what you are feeling is the normal postpartum adjustment that many fathers have to make. It may help to alleviate your frustration a bit by understanding some basic sexual differences between males and females. As you probably know, there are both mental and physical components of sex. In women, the mental component, or the feelings associated with sex, may be at least as important or more important than physical arousal. To a male, sex equals intercourse; to a female, this may not always be the case. The mental or nonsexual intercourse components of sex are often especially important to the postpartum mother. Many women are truly not ready for sexual intercourse until several months after birth. It seems that a mother's body is usually not ready until her mind is. Try these tips to woo back your wife: Don't pressure her into sexual intercourse too soon. Women whom we have interviewed on this subject relate that during the first month or two after birth they want to be held and loved, but feel they are not yet ready for intercourse. Go slowly. Even though the doctor may say your wife is ready for sexual intercourse at six weeks, she may not be ready. You may need to go through a progression similar to your premarital courtship. Your wife also feels the necessity to be reconnected sexually to you, but she probably needs a warm-up period of eye-to-eye contact, touching, caressing, and many "I care" messages before sexual intercourse can become fulfilling to her. Some caring fathers whom we have interviewed have described postpartum sexual relations as getting to know their wife all over again (See question 180).

182. *My wife is prone to depression, and after the birth of our first baby she was depressed for several weeks. We're expecting our next baby soon. Is there anything I can do to lessen her depression after birth? The previous experience was hard on both of us.*

Much of your wife's depression probably results from too many changes too soon. At no other time in a woman's life is she expected to do so much for so many with so little help. Here's what you can do:

1. Take a few weeks of paternity leave if possible. During this time, become chief of energy management in your household. Take over all those household energy-draining chores from your wife so that she has more left over to give to your baby and to herself.
2. Keep her nest clean and tidy. Postpartum mothers are especially sensitive to untidiness.
3. Take over the care of your older child as much as possi-

ble, since older siblings are particularly draining during the postpartum period.

4. Stand guard to protect your wife from unnecessary visitors and responsibilities. Take the phone off the hook while your wife and baby are sleeping and put a "do not disturb" sign on the door.

5. Keep harmony in the nest. Respect this early nesting instinct and do everything you can to keep others from disturbing the nest. Help with the household chores, and even do some cooking if you can. Serving your wife breakfast in bed is a sure winner. Ward off prophets of bad baby advice. Well-meaning friends, even your mother, may offer advice that shakes your wife's confidence. Postpartum mothers are particularly vulnerable to any remarks that suggests they may not be doing the right thing for their baby. Support your wife's confidence by giving her messages such as "You're doing the most important job in the world—mothering our baby."

6. Be sensitive. One of the most common complaints I receive in our practice is from mothers who feel that their husbands are not truly sensitive to their needs. A statement we often hear is: "I'd have to hit my husband over the head before he realized that I'm giving out." Don't take anything for granted in the postpartum mother. Ask your wife what she needs and what you can do to help. You may be surprised that little things which previously didn't matter now bother her greatly, such as leaving your shoes lying around the house. Developing the quality of paternal sensitivity is one of the greatest gifts you can give your wife—and your baby. (See question 180.)

183. *Our baby is one-month-old and my wife seems to be going downhill. She isn't taking care of herself and is getting downright sloppy about her grooming. What can I do to help?*

Many women suffer a body image problem after birth. They don't feel as attractive, and they don't feel they have the time for good grooming. This is part of the "my baby needs all of me" syndrome. This syndrome is not only a normal by-product of most committed mothers but may also be a sign of early burn-out. You may need to step in and insist that she take time out to take care of herself. Here are some specific tips on how to help your wife take better care of herself so that ultimately she can take better care of her baby: Make an appointment for her to have a facial or something she enjoys and drive her there. Be sure you market this as something for her good, and not yours, or she may fall victim of the common feeling of "I'm not as attractive to you as I used to be, so you want to fix me up."

It really helps if you try to share the overall care of your baby as much as possible. The more you prove yourself capable of sensitively caring for your baby, the more your wife will let go of her baby and take better care of herself. In our survey of the causes of mother burn-out we have found that one of the most precipitating causes is an uninvolved and insensitive husband.

184. *I really like to play with our six-month-old baby, but I can't seem to hold her attention as long as my wife can. I know you have several children. Can you give me some pointers?*

Who's better is not an issue in talking with and playing with your baby. You and your wife play differently with your baby, and babies profit from these different types of stimulation. The basic principal of holding a baby's attention is called *reciprocity*, and mothers are more natural at this art. Interesting studies in which mothers and babies were videotaped during conversations show that a mother takes time to listen to the baby's cues. Although the baby doesn't talk back, the mother naturally behaves as if the baby had responded to her. This turn-taking in conversations seems to develop more naturally between mothers and babies than between fathers and babies. Consequently, mothers develop a better holding power on the baby's attention. In addition to having a natural maternal instinct, another reason that mothers are able to hold their babies' attention longer is that they usually spend more time with them. Since fathers seldom have the luxury of spending long periods of unscheduled time with their babies, they are prone to overstimulating their infants. Perhaps you rush in and initiate a playful interaction too quickly. Your eagerness may agitate your baby and lessen her attention to you. Try the following tips to get your father–baby play off to the right start: Approach your baby gradually. This approach is called the *look, talk, and touch* sequence. First, establish eye contact. Then begin talking to your baby before you pick her up for play.

Another reason you may not be able to hold your baby's attention as well as your wife is because you may be in the mood to play but your baby isn't. Watch for cues that she is in a receptive state to play. This is probably when she is in a state of quiet alertness. Look for the following signs: her eyes are wide open and she seems generally attentive to what is going on around her, then she is in a good state to initiate play. If she seems sleepy or fussy, she is not in a state conducive to play. During the state of quiet alertness, watch for baby's cues that she wants to play—making eye contact with you, smiling, and reaching out to you with her hands. You can hold your baby's eye contact longer if you pick her up and hold her approximately twelve to eighteen inches from your face rather than bending over to talk to her while she is lying on her back in a crib. Watch, too, for "stop signs." When your baby begins a vacant stare and turns her eyes and head away from you, she may have had enough for now and you need to back off momentarily. Don't bombard your baby with too much for too long. Babies have short attention spans, often as little as one minute in a six-month-old. Short, frequent playful interactions are much better than forced, long interactions. Learning how to read your baby's interaction signals is part of your education as

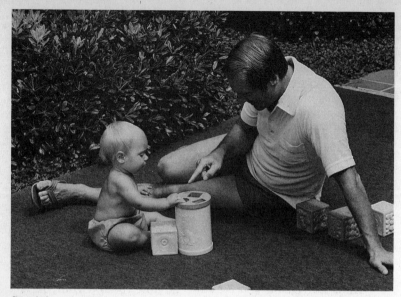

Special activities shared between father and baby can help the two to bond.

a father, which will eventually help you to read your whole baby—an important part in learning how to relate to and discipline your baby. Don't try to imitate the way in which your wife plays with your baby. Have confidence in your own way of relating to your baby, which is, again, not better, not worse, just different from your wife's. Babies thrive on this difference. You may also enrich your play activity by knowing what your baby's capabilities and preferences are at each developmental stage. (For more tips on interacting with your baby see books *Becoming a Father* and *Growing Together* in suggested library for parents, p. 283)

185. *I have recently married an older man. This is my first marriage, his second. He has two teenage children from a previous marriage. He wants to have a baby right away. What kind of father should I expect him to be?*

Most likely a good one, even better than in his first marriage. We call this "the second time around" syndrome.

More often than not, older fathers are more committed to fathering. In their first marriage, especially if they had children at a young age, they were busily climbing the professional ladder and were involved in many pursuits other than fathering. Older dads often realize what they missed with their first children, and having already climbed the professional ladder are now ready to settle down and be a committed father. It is heartwarming to see these dads attend their baby's well-baby checkups. They're as interested and knowledgeable about the baby as the mother. Your husband will probably be much more involved with the baby than some younger dads. Go for it!

186. *I've heard a lot about the importance of mothers bonding with their babies. We are expecting our first baby soon and I want to be part of the action too. Is father bonding important?*

Yes. Bonding is every bit as important for the father as for the mother. This bonding is important in a different way. Fifteen years ago when the concept of bonding became popular, most attention was given to mother–infant bonding. Father was given only a fine-print honorable mention, as it were. In the past few years the importance of father–baby bonding is just beginning to be studied and appreciated. In mother–infant bonding research the focus seems to be primarily on what the mother does for the infant. In father–infant bonding research the focus seems to be on what the infant does for the father. Researchers have coined the term *engrossment* to describe the good things that a newborn does for the father when the two are in touch with each other a lot during the newborn period. Dr. Martin Greenburg, in his book *The Birth of a Father*, describes engrossment (meaning "to make large") as a feeling fathers have that they have suddenly grown. They feel bigger, stronger, older, and more committed. Engrossment fits into a favorite theory of ours—a baby can bring out the best in the parents. This is certainly true of what a baby does to a father when the two form an attachment during the early weeks of life. The traditional stereotype of fathers as well-meaning but bumbling is only true of fathers who have not been given (or who have not taken) the opportunity to get to know their newborn. Studies have shown that fathers who are given the opportunity and are encouraged to take an active part in the care of their newborn become just as nurturing as mothers—not better at nurturing, not worse at nurturing, just different. One of the greatest of all maturing influences is that of a newborn baby on a grown man. Don't miss it! Get your hands on your baby right after birth. Hold and sing to your baby. That's how bonding begins. (See questions 178, 190 for other father bonding tips).

187. *I've heard a lot about a mother getting depressed after birth, but I'm starting to feel a bit depressed myself and our baby is only one month old. Can fathers experience postpartum depression too?*

Yes, but in a different way. Although fathers do not experience the physical and hormonal changes that mothers do, they have unique adjustment problems too. Your postpartum adjustment problems are probably due to your suddenly increased responsibilities and dramatic changes in life-style. You have another mouth to feed, your wife is never going to act the same or be the same (hopefully that's for the better), and you will probably never have as much time with your baby and wife as you want to have. Many fathers are overwhelmed by having to take care of a new baby and be a husband to their wives—who need a bit of mothering themselves. The demands of fathering a baby and mothering a mother may be too much too soon and result in depression. It is an awesome responsibility to hold a major part of the outcome of another human being in your hands. It helps to focus more on the joys of fathering rather than just the responsibilities; realize the fun you are now having and will continue to have with your baby—this fun will change at every stage of your baby's development, and your development. If you allow it to flow naturally, your baby will give to you as much as you give to him. Also, don't let yourself be so preoccupied with the things you must get for your baby that you lose sight of your interactions with him that will profit him more than the toys you buy. Give of yourself. It's much better and less expensive.

188. *I will soon become a grandfather for the first time. My daughter wants to stay home, but has to go back to work after a few months because her husband is still a student and they need the money. I want to help, but I don't want to interfere. Is it right to give them some money?*

Yes. Perhaps this situation is best illustrated by relating a story about one of our patients. Jack, a stockbroker friend, would frequently call with the advice, "Doc, I've got a good investment for you." Shortly after Jack became a grandfather for the first time and his daughter was in a similar working dilemma as yours, I called him and said, "Jack, I've got the best investment tip you've ever heard." I went on to advise him that the best investment into his grandchild's future would be to give or loan the new couple enough money to allow his grandchild to have the best start in life— the interaction with a full-time mother. He thanked me and made the investment. There is a historical precedent for this type of investment. In many cultures it used to be and sometimes still is customary to give an inheritance to couples when they became new parents rather than after the death of a grandparent. Financial pressures are one of the greatest stresses on today's young parents. Grandparents can help a lot. If financial assistance is not possible, grandparents can offer to baby-sit. Mothers returning to work feel much better about their situation when they trust their substitute care giver.

189. *We have one of those high-need babies, as you call them. She needs to be held a lot and I try to help my wife* *as much as possible, but I just can't seem to get the hang of it. She squirms and arches whenever I try to pick her up. Any tips?*

Don't always imitate your wife's methods of carrying your baby. Fathers hold their babies differently, and babies profit from this difference. Here are some time-tested favorite holding patterns for fathers.

1. The football hold. Drape your baby tummy down over your forearm like a football, her neck in the crook of your arm and the diaper area in your hand. Grasp the diaper area firmly in your hand and gently press the base of the palm of your hand against your baby's tense abdomen.

2. The neck nestle. This is one of my favorites, and actually works better for males. Nestle your baby's head against the curvature of your neck, allowing your chin to rest on top of her head. Gently push her head against your Adam's apple (the bulge of your voice box in the front part of your neck). Babies hear with the vibration of their skull bones in addition to their eardrums. Sing a droning song, such as "Old Man River," in a deep male voice. The vibrations of your voice box and jawbones against your baby's thin skull will often lull a fussy baby right to sleep. An added attraction of the neck nestle is that your baby will feel the warm air from your nose on her scalp. Experienced mothers relate that breathing on their babies' faces or heads calms them. Fathers may have a "magic breath" all their own.

3. The front bend. Fussy babies often settle better in the bent position as if this relaxes the spinal muscles and therefore the whole body. With your baby facing you, flex her legs against your chest, and support her back with one hand and the nape of her neck with the other. When baby is bent in a *C* position, she often settles better and expels more gas. If she squirms in the back-forward position, turn her around, still bent, and let her face forward, allowing her back and head to rest against

your chest while holding her outstretched legs over your folded arms.

5. The shoulder ride. Around six months a baby's head control has developed enough so she can sit erect and enjoy riding on your shoulders. Babies seem to like this riding position around five or six months because their hands, head, and back are less restrained and they have a three-hundred-and-sixty-degree view of their world.

6. Choose the right baby carrier. Most fathers do not feel comfortable with many of the baby carriers on the market because there are too many straps and buckles for the impatient male. We have found that the sling-type carrier works best for men because it is much easier to adjust. It is frustrating to pick up a fussy baby and try to make many adjustments in a carrier that has been previously adjusted to conform to your wife's body. This is called the art of wearing your baby—and it's as important for fathers to learn as for mothers. (See questions 37, 38.)

190. *I love to touch and massage our baby's skin. I've noticed that he responds differently to my touch than to my wife's. Is this my imagination or can six-month-old babies really feel the difference?*

Yes, they can—and it's a good difference to feel. Mothers and fathers intuitively touch and massage their babies differently. Mothers tend to use more of their fingertips and a lighter stroke, whereas fathers tend to use their whole hand. Try the following massage tips: Place your baby, unclothed, on a soft surface such as a lambskin. Be sure the room is warm and your hands are warm (immerse your hands in warm water and dry them before starting, or rub them together vigorously to increase the heat to your palms). Warm the oil by placing a small amount in your hands and vigorously rubbing your hands together. Babies like wide, circular strokes. Start with the neck and then gradually do the limbs, stroking from the shoulder all the way to the tips of the fingers and from the groin to the soles of his feet.

Tense babies have tense limbs. When you see your baby's fists gradually unfolding and his limbs dangling limply from his sides, you know that your soothing massage is getting through to him.

191. *I love to play with our one-year-old baby, but sometimes she gets bored and so do I. What toys should I buy?*

Toys are not always the answers to having playful fun. It is what you do with those toys that counts. Play is most fun and most sustained if you use toys and interactions that best fit your baby's developmental skills at a certain age. The prime developmental skills of one-year-olds are: an ability to sit erect for long periods of time, crawling, and short-term memory of disappearing objects. Based upon these developmental skills, here are some time-tested favorites for the one-year-old: Roll out the carpet. A baby's attention in any play activity is better sustained by having a setting event that is unique to father play—something you do that no other family member does. A game that our one-year-old, Matthew, and I enjoyed is what I call, "Roll out the carpet." Buy a piece of indoor-outdoor carpet approximately six-by-ten feet, (usually available as an inexpensive remnant at a carpet store). Leave the carpet rolled up on your patio next to a basket full of toys. In rainy or cold weather, a basement or garage is an alternative play area. When your baby sees you roll out the carpet and sit down, her memory clicks into a groove that she is being set up for a fun play time. She will then probably crawl or walk toward the basket full of toys. She is most likely to play with the toys longer if she has picked them up herself.

Play pitch and go fetch. Use a large foam ball that your baby can hold with both hands. Roll the ball toward her and hold your hands up for her to throw the ball back to you. Don't expect too many strikes at this age. Ping-pong balls are also a favorite ball at this stage. Sing while you play. As you roll the ball, sing, "Get the ball." Your baby at one year can understand a one-step request. After she gets the

ball, follow with "Throw to Dad." Accompany your verbal
gestures with throwing gestures, for many one-year-olds
need gestures to help them decode what you want.

Playing with blocks is a perennial favorite, and the older
the baby, the larger the blocks. Babies love to tower blocks
with dad and then topple their tower.

Hide-and-seek around the sofa is another favorite, with
dad crawling around and hiding behind the sofa, periodically
popping his head up from different places exclaiming,
"Where's Dad?" (It helps to intersperse with "Here I am"
as you pop your head up again.)

Between nine months and a year babies love container
play—putting small objects into large boxes and dumping
them out again. One of the feelings that a father must
overcome is the impression that you are wasting time with
this simple play and should be doing something important
instead. While stacking blocks may not be as important to
you as building bridges, it is to your baby. Not only is she
learning, you are learning as well: how to relate to your
baby. The more you learn to relate to her in simple things,
the easier you will form more complex relations later on.
(For additional father play tips see suggested Library for
Parents, P. 283.)

192. *My wife is still nursing our two-year-old. She holds
him a lot, doesn't let him cry, and still treats him like a
baby, although I think he should be starting to grow up by
now. I guess I have a real fear of him growing up to be a
sissy or even homosexual. Should I be afraid of this?*

No. Appropriate nurturing of a toddler, as it seems your
wife is doing, does not cause homosexuality or effeminate
behavior in males. In fact, studies have shown that sex-role
identity problems may be caused more by what a father
does *not* do rather than by what a mother does. Inadequate
fathering seems to be more of a contributing factor to homosexuality in boys and girls than inadequate mothering. Since

this does seem to be a concern to you, there are some things you can do.

While we don't always know why people are homosexual, studies have shown that homosexuality is more common in families with a weak, uninvolved father and a dominant mother, plus a weak husband–wife relationship. Allow your wife to nurture your two-year-old as she is doing, but complement her nurturing with your own brand of nurturing. Children who grow up regarding their father as not only a fair disciplinarian but a sensitive nurturer tend to have the healthiest sex identities. The best way to alleviate your concerns is to love your wife as a caring and supportive mate, allow her to nurture your baby according to her own mothering intuition, and balance her type of nurturing by providing much of your own. (See question 193 for suggestions on how fathers can develop healthy attitudes toward sexuality.)

193. *Our two-and-a-half-year-old son plays with dolls. This bothers me. I want our boys to grow up to be real boys and our girls to be real girls. Any suggestions?*

Defining masculinity and femininity is difficult without succumbing to cultural stereotyping. We are led to believe that the term masculine means assertive, decisive, physical, deliberate, and logical. Femininity is often associated with sensitivity, warmth, expressiveness, and ego-building qualities (used to capture the male's attention, of course!). Perhaps it is more accurate to state that one set of traits predominates in a healthy masculine or feminine identity, but that each sex possesses some or all of the qualities in both categories.

It is fair to say that fathers are more concerned about masculine and feminine behavior than mothers. A father may give a boy a football expecting him to kick it and give a daughter a doll expecting her to cuddle it. When the son cuddles the football and the daughter kicks the doll, the father's well laid plans go astray. Mothers may give dolls or stuffed animals to cuddle and nurture to either boys or girls. You should realize that the fact that you and your wife approach the teaching of sex roles differently can result in a healthy balance for your child. Fathers seem to steer the child toward predominantly one sex role, whereas mothers allow the child to adopt some qualities associated with both sexes. Like so many aspects of parenting, the key issue here is balance. Let your little boy play with dolls as well as other toys. Boys need to develop tenderness too.

194. *I am a new father and already I have money worries. I want to be the only breadwinner in the family and my wife wants to be a full-time mother, but I worry about making ends meet. Any suggestions?*

Your concerns about being the breadwinner are a normal part of the profession of fathering, and apparently you take this profession seriously. You have chosen the traditional family economic structure with the father as the only bread-winner—a decision which is becoming more and more difficult for many families in today's world. Here are some suggestions to help you juggle family finances, your job and time with your family: Verbalize your worries to your wife so that she can understand and help you make some basic financial decisions. It helps when husband and wife are in agreement about where to cut financial corners. Basically you both are making the decision that family relationships are more important than material things. Decide together which things you can temporarily do without, which you must have, and how much you can afford.

Take the leadership role in the family by conveying to your wife that you feel that it is more important that you have time with your family than to take a second job or work many longer hours to earn extra income. This is a trade-off that you are asking your wife to accept. While you may have less money, you are asking your wife to value your role as an active participant in child care and not only as a breadwinner. In our experience most mothers place a higher value on their having an involved father than on bringing home a higher paycheck. Part of your growth and development as a new father is to learn to balance your financial commitment to your family with the commitment of yourself to your child. If there is no way you can make ends meet with you as the only breadwinner, then consider having your wife help supplement the income by finding a way to work at home. The possibilities are endless; a few ideas to get you thinking are child care, telephone soliciting, typing, word processing, catering, tutoring, and home businesses such as mail order or sewing. (A good reference text which discusses many alternatives to working outside the home and ways to earn extra income at home is the book *The Heart Has Its Own Reasons*, published by La Leche League International, Franklin Park, Ill., 1986.)

195. *My job requires me to travel a great deal. I don't like it, but I'm committed to finishing a project which requires me to be away one or two days a week for the next few months. We have a one-year-old and we're very close. What can I do to maintain this attachment even though I have to travel?*

Your dilemma is shared by thousands of traveling fathers who miss being with their babies, yet realize their important role as the breadwinner. As one traveling father of a large family put it, "Someone has to fund this operation!" Try leaving as much of yourself behind as possible and use all the latest technology to maintain contact with your wife and baby while you are away. Leave tape recordings of yourself singing a bedtime song to your baby and little father-love messages. Be sure to use phrases and songs that your baby associates with you. Leave photographs of yourself. During our recent baby's first year I hung an eight-by-ten black-and-white photograph of myself on the side of her changing table so that she would at least see a picture of me if I couldn't be there. Mothers have told us that they often bring out the pictures and tape recordings of dad (audio and video) during those moments of the day when the baby seems particularly fussy. Bringing back memories of dad seems to soothe the baby during a fussy period, as if she reflects upon the memory of a special person who is missing. Call and talk to your child frequently, especially before bedtime. When she gets older you may even call this the "surprise call." Telling a bedtime story by phone is a winner. In fact, it is quite common for mothers to get a bit fussy when dad is away because one of their major support people is not around. Don't be disappointed if your baby gives you a temporary cold shoulder when you return. Babies feel a mixture of anger and confusion about dad being away and may need some time to adjust to your return. To smooth your reentry, don't immediately come on too strong but gradually re-bond with your baby by clicking her into one of her favorite fun activities with you. Hold her in one of her favorite ways and sing one of her favorite songs. Soon you will strike a familiar note and have a happy reunion.

6

ILLNESSES,
ACCIDENTS,
AND PREVENTIVE
MEDICINE

The medical advice in this section on parenting your baby through illness and accident prevention is based upon our experience in nearly twenty years of pediatric practice, our experience as parents of seven children, and advice from trusted colleagues. We also include the most up-to-date advice from current medical journals. The answers in this chapter are formulated to help parents recognize early signs of illness, and then by knowing what to watch for to determine if an illness is or is not serious—when to worry, when not to worry. We want this chapter to take much of the anxiety out of caring for a sick child and teach you how to become more comfortable in parenting your sick child. Many of the answers tell you when to call your baby's doctor and help you communicate more accurately with health care professionals. Many practical self-help remedies are sprinkled throughout the answers to help you be your child's home doctor. We purposely avoid questionable forms of treatment, since children are too valuable and parents too vulnerable to try treatments which

176

have not been proven safe and effective. Enjoy this chapter
as you strive to keep your child safe and healthy.

196. *Our six-month-old wakes up with a runny nose and
watery eyes. We do have a lot of allergies in the family. Do
you think our baby might have allergies too?*

Yes. The clue here is that he wakes up stuffy. The first
place to start helping your baby is his bedroom and sleeping
environment. Perhaps the most allergenic environment in
the whole world is a child's bedroom, full of stuffed animals,
feather pillows, and all the places dust collects. De-fuzz your
baby's sleeping environment. Remove stuffed animals, the
family dog or cat, and any other potential dust collectors.
Often this will be enough to alleviate your baby's symptoms.
If he still wakes up stuffy, get non-allergenic bed coverings
and mattress. In severe cases you may need to remove the
carpet from the bedroom and place washable throw rugs on
a wooden or tile floor. Consider a change in laundry soap.
Wash new bed clothing and sleepwear through several wash
cycles to remove the normal fabric fuzz. Also, do not allow
anyone to smoke in the house. Cigarette smoke is a common
nasal irritant to babies. If you use heating or air conditioning, clean and replace the air filter frequently. If your baby
seems to be very allergenic, try an electronic air filter in
his bedroom. Molds and mildews which collect in damp walls
(especially if you use a humidifier or vaporizer frequently)
may also be a bedroom allergen.

197. *Our one-year-old seems to constantly have a runny
nose, and I can't tell whether it is an allergy or a cold.
What is the difference?*

Sometimes it is very difficult to tell a runny nose caused by
an allergy from that caused by a cold. Allergies are caused
by a foreign substance in the air which triggers the mucus-
producing cells in the lining of your child's nose. A cold is
caused by a germ which can infect these same cells and

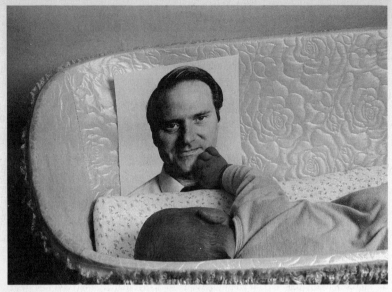

Absent fathers can leave mementos for their babies.

produce mucus. Here are the usual differences: The fluid from an allergic runny nose is usually clear, watery, and associated with other signs of allergy such as puffy, watery eyes, family history of allergies, seasonal variation or some identifiable trigger which causes your child's nose to run more. On the other hand, the nasal discharge from a cold tends to be thicker and yellower. A cold is usually associated with other signs of an infection, including yellow drainage from the eyes, a low-grade fever, and a cough. A cold tends to get steadily worse over a few days and then get better. Sometimes a nasal discharge can begin as an allergy, but the allergic fluid serves as a culture medium for the growth of germs, and before long, an infection is present in addition to the allergy.

198. *Our two-and-a-half-year-old has had a lingering cough for the past six weeks. She doesn't have a fever and does not act sick. The cough is mainly a nuisance that* *wakes her up and interferes with her play. Our doctor has checked her and doesn't find anything wrong. Should I be concerned?*

The main question to ask yourself when your child is sick with a cold is "How much is it bothering her?" If she eats well, sleeps well, doesn't have a fever, plays well, and the cold is just a noisy nuisance, then it is probably a lingering virus which will go away with a tincture of time and without prescription medication. If your child's cough is keeping her awake at night and interfering with her enjoyment of play in the daytime, you might consider the following: She could be allergic to something in her bedroom, such as dust collectors including stuffed animals, feather pillows, and all the fuzzy stuff that commonly resides in a child's bedroom. De-fuzz her sleeping environment. In addition, do some detective work to see if there are any new allergens in her environment, such as cigarette smoke, new foods, new toys, new laundry soap, or house plants.

A subtle cause of chronic coughs in children is a sinus infection. The sinuses are small cavities around the eyes and alongside the nose in which fluid often accumulates during a cold. When your child lies down during sleep, the postnasal drip may cause her to cough. Take your child back to your doctor to check for a possible sinus infection. If the cough has lingered on and is bothering your child increasingly, a chest X ray may be necessary.

199. *Our two-year-old gets a lot of colds. When should I take him to a doctor, and when will the cold go away by itself?*

Look for three signs: what comes out of your child's nose, the characteristics of his face, and his general behavior. If the discharge from his nose is clear and watery, he still has a normal pink and sparkly countenance, and he is generally happy even though he coughs and sneezes, he probably just has a cold, which will go away with good nasal hygiene and time. If the nasal discharge becomes increasingly thick, yellow, and green (the runny nose becomes a snotty nose); your child's facial appearance becomes peaked (pale, droopy, discharging eyes) and his behavior goes from happy to cranky, especially if all these symptoms are accompanied by a fever and pain in the throat or ears, you should take your child to the doctor.

200. *Our one-year-old is prone to ear infections. I'm in the doctor's office every six weeks for antibiotics. What can I do to prevent them?*

One of the most common causes of recurrent ear infections is allergies. Some allergens, either in the environment or the diet, trigger the release of fluid into the middle ear, similar to the way in which fluid is released in an allergic runny nose. The fluid serves as a culture medium encouraging the growth of bacteria in the middle ear behind the eardrum, resulting in a middle-ear infection. The antibiotics kill the germs, but the fluid remains, soon becoming reinfected and resulting in another trip to the doctor. The key is to get rid of both the germs and the fluid. Start by getting rid of the most common allergens, something in your child's immediate environment or in her diet. Get rid of all fuzzy things in her sleeping environment; including stuffed animals, feather pillows, any dust collectors in the bed or bedroom. Keep your child away from cigarette smoke and remove all potentially allergic plants and animals from her immediate environment. If you do not notice any improvement, the allergen could be in her diet. The most common food allergens are: dairy products, wheat, citrus, nuts, and eggs. Keep an allergy diary to pinpoint your child's allergy. Mothers are usually good detectives. If you are still unable to identify the offending allergen but suspect that allergens are the culprit, consult an allergist.

201. *Our two-year-old has had one ear infection after another. Our neighbor's child had the same problem, but is* *now a lot better after having had tubes put in his ears. What is this operation and do you think it might help our child?*

Possibly. This operation, called tympanostomy, is the insertion of tubes through the eardrums. Your child is given a light general anesthesia, and an ENT specialist places tiny plastic or metal tubes about the size of a pencil lead through the eardrums. These tubes "ventilate" the middle-ear cavity, allowing the fluid to drain out so that it cannot become infected. Although this operation is very effective in many children with recurrent ear infections, it does not always work and is not always necessary. There are three levels in treating children's ear infections: Level one includes the child who gets an occasional ear infection, is treated for seven to ten days with antibiotics, and is reexamined and treated until the infection is completely cleared. If the child starts getting ear infections more frequently and they are lasting longer, then the child is placed on level two treatment regimen. A thorough allergic investigation is performed to determine whether or not allergies are the cause of fluid in the middle ear. The child is placed on a daily dose of a mild antibiotic such as a sulfa medication, as part of a treatment called a preventive regimen. The use of daily antibiotics in a preventive way is a relatively new treatment, and it has been very effective for many children. In this way, your child maintains a constant level of the antibiotic in the blood stream, which keeps the fluid in the middle ear from becoming infected. Often, a daily dose of a mild antibiotic is much easier on your child's system than periodic stronger antibiotics. This same medication has been given daily to children for twenty years to prevent rheumatic fever and has no apparent side effects. This prevention regimen is prescribed for three to six months, especially during the winter months. It sounds like your child is a candidate for this prevention regimen.

A small percentage of children fail this level two prevention regimen and still get recurrent middle-ear infections. These children are candidates for level three treatment—tympanostomy tubes. It is important to give your child an adequate trial of the prevention regimen before jumping unnecessarily into the operation.

202. *Our two-year-old daughter gets a lot of ear infections, and they always seem to come on at night. I hate to bother our doctor all the time at night. Is there anything I can do to relieve the pain until I can take her in to the doctor the next morning?*

Thank you for being so considerate of your doctor. The reason that children complain more of sore ears at night than during the day is because when your child lies flat, the infected fluid presses on her eardrum. When she is upright, usually during the day, the fluid does not cause as much pressure on the eardrum and therefore does not cause as much pain. Here are some suggestions on helping your child, and your doctor, get through the night: Prop your child upright on a couple of pillows. Give her age- and weight-appropriate doses of either acetaminophen or aspirin. (If using acetaminophen you can safely double the recommended dosage for two doses given three hours apart. (See question 218 for discussion of acetominophen.) To relieve the pain, warm some cooking oil such as corn oil or olive oil in a bowl set in warm water and instill four or five drops of warm oil in the canal of the hurting ear. Encourage your child to turn her head so that the sore ear is upright. This position allows the warm oil to reach and soothe the infected eardrum at the bottom of the canal. Sometimes a child may wake up during the night with a sore ear but seem better in the morning, and the parents feel that their child didn't really have an ear infection and not bother to take her to the doctor. This assumption is wrong. A child with an ear infection commonly feels better upon awakening simply because she is upright and there's less pressure on the middle ear. Always take your child to the doctor if you have any suspicion that she has an ear infection.

203. *My child gets a lot of ear infections, but I'm confused about the difference between outer-ear infections and middle-ear infections. What is the difference?*

Outer-ear infection means an inflammation of the lining of the ear canal in front of the eardrum. With these infections, the child winces with pain when you wiggle the infected ear. This type of infection is usually caused by an irritation to the lining of the ear canal such as that caused by swimming. Outer-ear infections are sometimes called "swimmer's ear." These infections are seldom serious, do not permanently impair the hearing, and can be treated with antibiotic ear drops. Middle-ear infection, on the other hand, means an infection behind the eardrum. If not properly treated, this type of an infection may impair the hearing. Middle-ear infection causes intense pain and is usually not aggravated by wiggling the ear. These infections require more careful treatment and follow-up by the physician.

204. *Our two-year-old gets a great many colds. Would it help to keep him indoors when he gets sick, or should I let him go outside?*

By all means let him go outside. Fresh air and sunshine are good for a child. Going out in cold air does not cause colds. One of the main reasons why children get more colds in the wintertime is that they tend to be kept indoors and in closer contact with each other. The closer contact, not the cold weather, aggravates colds.

205. *I provide day care in my home and the children range in age from three months to three years. Because their mothers have to work, they sometimes drop their children off even when they have colds. I want to be sensitive to these mothers, yet I feel that I also have a responsibility to keep the colds from spreading to the other children. When should I insist that mothers keep sick children at home?*

This indeed is a dilemma, especially if the mothers have to work. Missing a day's work because of a child who is not particularly sick but is possibly contagious is a hardship on some families. Try the following policies: If the child has a watery runny nose, no fever, and doesn't look or act particularly sick, then she probably just has a cold and may safely come into day care. If she has a persistently snotty nose (thick, yellow drainage), looks peaked, and has a fever and cough, then she should not be allowed to communicate with the other children. If the mother herself seems in doubt as to whether the child is contagious, encourage her to ask her doctor, or best of all, to bring a note from the doctor. If the child does not appear very sick but you are uncertain as to whether or not she is contagious, a compromise solution is to isolate her in a room for a day to determine how sick she really is. By the end of the day you will know whether or not she is sick enough to continue in day care or should be at home.

206. *Our one-and-a-half-year-old is on antibiotics much of the time, and gets diarrhea as a result. How can we prevent this?*

In addition to killing harmful bacteria, antibiotics also kill certain desirable bacteria that reside in the intestines. These provide beneficial services to the intestines in return for a place to live. This is the normal ecology of the gut. One of the common favorable bacteria that is killed by antibiotics is the Lactobacillus bifidus. You can minimize the diarrhea from the antibiotics by giving your child a daily dose of one capful or one tablet of L. bifidus (available in refrigerated form in most nutrition stores). Babies also commonly get diaper rashes during antibiotic therapy because their stools become very acidic, giving a reddened, burned appearance to the skin of the diaper area. In addition to giving your child L. bifidus, a baking soda bath (a tablespoon of baking soda in a tiny tub of water) should soothe the rash.

207. *Our one-year-old baby has sensitive intestines. Every time he gets a cold, he gets diarrhea. What should I do and when should I worry about the problem?*

As a general guide, no weight loss; no worry. Children often have looser stools than usual during most colds. If your baby is not losing much weight quickly, you don't have to worry. As a general guide, you should be concerned when your child loses more than five percent of his body weight (a weight loss of one pound in a twenty-pound child). If he has lost this amount gradually over a period of about a week, the problem is not serious; however, a quick weight loss from profuse diarrhea over a day or two is more worrisome. Remember, during most diarrhea illnesses, the lining of the intestines is injured and needs a long time to heal. A period of several weeks is usually necessary, during which time your child's stools may be looser than usual although he appears well. If your child is not losing weight and does not appear ill, a change in diet is usually not necessary. If the diarrhea seems to be worsening take your child off foods which may aggravate the symptoms, including dairy products and fatty foods. You do not have to stop breastfeeding if your child has diarrhea. A change of formula or dilution of the present amount of formula may be necessary, as well as a bland diet of rice cereal and bananas for a day or two. Here's a dietary tip on returning him to his regular diet: As your child's stools become more solid, so can his diet. If he seems to be losing more weight or becoming sicker, call your doctor.

208. *Our two-year-old frequently gets colds and ear infections, and needs a lot of antibiotics. I worry about giving her so much medicine. Are antibiotics really safe?*

Yes. Children get two general types of germs—viruses and bacteria. Viral infections usually do not require antibiotics; bacterial infections do. The main judgment your doctor tries to make when examining your child is what type of infection she has. Every medicine has what we call a benefit–risk ratio, meaning that the benefits of the medicine far outweigh the risks of taking it or the risk of what would happen if it were not given. In the case of bacterial infections, the risk of your child getting much sicker without antibiotic treatment is much greater than the risk of a potentially harmful effect of the antibiotic. In general, antibiotics have a high benefit–risk ratio, meaning that they have few side effects if used wisely. A small number of children are allergic to antibiotics, and antibiotics often cause temporary diarrhea. However, in nearly twenty years of pediatric practice, we have seen many more problems with the underuse of antibiotics than with the overuse. Trust your doctor's judgment if she says the child needs an antibiotic.

Sometimes when a doctor initially sees a child it may be unclear whether the child has a bacterial or a viral infection. If she suspects a viral infection, an antibiotic usually will not be prescribed. It is important for you to check back with your doctor should your child's illness get worse. Then your doctor can reevaluate the initial judgment as more definite signs and symptoms appear.

209. *Our two-year-old just won't take medicine. The hassle of giving it to him sometimes seems worse than his illness. Any tips on handling this struggle?*

Here are some tips that creative parents have shared with us concerning their successful negotiations with reluctant medicine takers. Most medicines come in different flavors and are made by different manufacturers. If your child needs a certain generic type of medicine, experiment with different brands to find the one that is most palatable for your child. Remember that brand name and ask for the same one the next time. In general, do not put medicines in a glass of juice or milk unless this practice is approved by your doctor. Use a calibrated syringe instead of a spoon to measure appropriate dosages. The syringe should be calibrated in cc's or ml's. Five cc's or ml's equals one teaspoon.

If you have more than one child, try the following trick. Your two-year-old will not want to be left out of anything good. Pass a spoonful of medicine around to the other children and have them pretend to swallow it, after which they should give an approving yum-yum sign. Your toddler will not want to miss out on the "goodies." Some children are better pill takers than liquid swallowers. Some medicines come in better-tasting chewable forms, even for the two-year-old. If your child simply will not swallow an unpalatable liquid, ask for the medication in capsule or pill form, crunch it up in a spoon, adding a bit of camouflaging with his favorite food. Play creative medicine-taking games such as the following: The spoonful of medicine flies like an airplane and lands in baby's open mouth. Run and bite—toddler takes a short run and makes a quick "pit stop" to take his spoonful of medicine. Babies often "forget" that they are really taking medicine if it is given during part of a play activity. Sometimes bribery is warranted, as in the Mary Poppins technique of "A spoonful of sugar helps the medicine go down." Use a piece of sugarless candy or a nutritious cookie. The use of hand puppets may also entice the reluctant medicine taker. Pretend to give the medicine to the open mouth of the hand puppet, or have the puppet ask your baby to take his medicine. Most two-year-olds can't be fooled with this, but they like to play the game anyway. As you are marketing the medicine, be sure to give affirming cues to your child such as "Medicine is *good* for baby." If all else fails, obtain the medicine in pill form, crush, and make a paste out of the pill. With your fingertip full of the medicine paste, place a small amount at a time on the inside of your toddler's cheek. Even though many of them don't often like to take medicine, they may trust this approach.

210. *I am a safety-conscious parent, and I'm really afraid that our nine-month-old will get hurt. Can you give me some accident-prevention tips for this stage?*

A general principal of accident prevention which will carry

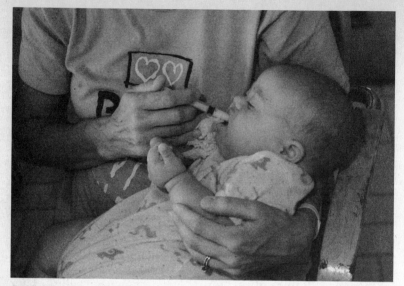

Babies can be very reluctant to take their medicine. Be sure to ask your doctor about how and when to give medicine, especially if special equipment is involved.

you through all ages is the following: Determine what your baby's new developmental skills are and, consequently, what accidents could result from her using these new skills. In the nine-to-twelve month stage a baby develops two main skills which may lead to accidents: thumb and forefinger pickup, and pulling up from crawling to standing. Because of their newly acquired skill of thumb and forefinger pickup, babies are fascinated by small, pellet-like objects that are commonly found on the floor. If you have an older sibling or there are toddlers or preschool age children around the house, be sure to counsel them not to leave small objects on the floor that a baby may pick up and choke on. Avoid toys which have small parts that a baby may pick off and put in his mouth.

Progressing from crawling to standing to walking also creates a variety of accident-prone situations. On your hands and knees, make a safety patrol around the house, looking for potential safety hazards from your baby's viewpoint. Look for objects that she could fall against, such as sharp table corners, fireplace bricks, chair corners, or any other sharp edges protruding from furniture. Cover these potential hazards with soft padding. We have used adhesive-backed weather stripping to line sharp edges that the beginning walker might fall against. Other common accidents at this stage include: grabbing accidents—hot coffee and breakable glass; high-chair accidents—crawling out of and falling from the high chair; and electrical burns—poking an exploring finger into electric outlets. These accidents can be prevented by anticipatory vigilance: Always fasten safety straps in high chairs, never put breakable objects or hot drinks within a baby's reach, and use safety plugs in electric outlets. Remember that babies are highly motivated to practice a newly acquired development skill, which leaves them particularly accident prone during the transition from one developmental stage to another.

211. *We have a nine-month-old who really enjoys his walker, but I have heard that walkers may not be safe or may delay motor development. Is this true?*

We have two concerns about walkers. They are potentially unsafe and they may interfere with a baby's normal development. Babies must learn to use their body parts in the normal progression that they were designed to follow. We do not advise parents to use walkers or any other devices which encourage babies to rely on outside assistance for locomotion rather than on their own creativity or initiative. We believe that babies are designed to progress from sitting to standing to walking by experimenting on their own and not with the aid of wheels or devices. In all but the most impulsive infants, mental and motor abilities develop in parallel. A baby's inability to think through a situation prevents him from using his newly found motor skills in situations he is not yet able to handle. Walkers may give babies motor skills that will get them into situations that they are not yet able to cope with mentally. A baby's normal motor development progresses from head to feet. Walkers reverse this process by giving the legs abilities that the head is not yet ready for. This reversal may produce accidents. Most babies do enjoy walkers, however, and brief spells of supervised walker play are probably all right. Spending a lot of time in a walker is not advisable. If you do use a walker, observe the following safety suggestions:

1. Walkers tip easily. Be sure the wheel base is much larger than the frame that holds the baby. A properly designed walker should not tip when he leans over the side.
2. Be sure the wheels are sturdy. Flimsy wheels may bend, allowing the walker to tip.
3. Remove throw rugs and other obstacles which may become entangled in the wheels and cause the walker to tip.
4. Do not allow walkers near stairs. Do not rely on stair gates. An impulsive infant may get up enough momentum to cruise right through the gate.
5. Be sure all coiled springs and hinges are encased in protective covers. Avoid the older X-frame walkers which can pinch a baby's fingers.

212. *Our ten-month-old gets into things from morning till night. We are considering buying a playpen. Are playpens a good idea for the crawling age?*

In general, it is good for a baby to get into things, as long as the normal curious exploration is done under parental supervision. If you have a situation in which you cannot watch your baby at all times, she may have an accident and a playpen is therefore advisable. Mothers who work at home or take their babies to work find playpens indispensable. When you shop for a playpen, observe the following safety tips:

1. Make sure the netting is small enough so that it cannot catch on the buttons of the child's clothing.
2. Avoid strings or cords that are longer than twelve inches and dangle from the sides of the playpen or from toys inside.

3. Remove large toys or boxes from inside the playpen that the baby could use to climb out.
4. Cover any exposed nuts or bolts. Secure latching mechanisms that could act like scissors and pinch a baby's fingers.
5. Be sure the playpen you buy meets the Juvenile Products Manufacturers Safety Standards (the JPMA seal should be affixed to the product stating that it has the association's approval).

Unless you need a playpen in particular circumstances, we generally discourage its use. Restricting a baby's exploratory environment may restrict her curiosity, which is a prime motivator to learn new developmental skills.

213. *Our baby loves toys and so do I. We are a safety-conscious family and want to choose safe toys. Any suggestions?*

Here are some tips for choosing safe toys: Avoid sharp-edged toys. Avoid those with small, removable objects (beads, buttons, etc.) which could be swallowed. Avoid the small metal or plastic parts that produce the noise in squeak toys, as they can come loose and be swallowed. Be sure blocks and the heads of rattles are too large to swallow. The smallest diameter of block and rattle toys should be no less than 1–3/8 inch. Toys should fit your child's age and temperament. If he is a thrower, get him soft, lightweight toys. Avoid missile-type toys (darts and arrows) which can cause eye injuries. Many accidents occur when a younger child uses toys meant for an older sibling. Avoid any string longer than eight inches attached to a toy, mobile, pacifier, or clothing. Strings can strangle. Put toy shelves in most rooms to encourage your child not to leave his toys lying where someone else could trip over them. Even infants as young as nine months enjoy toy shelves.

Toy and baby product manufacturers are becoming increasingly more safety-conscious, mainly due to public and government pressure. Be sure you read the instructions on the use of the toys and baby products you buy, use them only for the purpose for which they are intended, and observe the safety precautions advised by the manufacturer. If you have questions about the safety of a particular toy or baby product, information may be obtained from the following sources: Consumer Product Safety Commission, Washington, D.C. 20207, or call toll free 800-638-2772. In Canada contact: Department of Product Safety, 1410 Stanley Street, Montreal, Quebec H3A1P8, 514-283-2825.

214. *Our seven-month-old is restless in her tub-like car seat, and we think she is ready for a larger one. How old should a baby be before parents install a regular car seat and face it forward?*

Most car-seat manufacturers recommend switching from a rear-facing, tub-like carrier to the front-facing, semi-upright carrier when the baby's weight reaches between seventeen and twenty pounds. Some car seats accommodate both front and back facing positions in the same seat. Most babies reach that weight at eight to twelve months of age. Be sure to buy a carrier which meets government testing and safety standards. Information on car-safety devices can be obtained in a pamphlet from the American Academy of Pediatrics. Send a stamped, self-addressed envelope requesting the 1989 Family Shopping Guide to Infant/Child Safety Seats to: American Academy of Pediatrics, P.O. Box 927, Oak Grove Village, IL 60009-0927.

215. *We have a backyard pool and want to teach our one-year-old baby to swim. I've heard a lot of controversy about whether or not it is safe for babies to be in swimming pools or even if they should learn to swim at such an early age. What is your advice?*

Since you have a backyard pool, you definitely need to teach your baby to swim, in addition to taking the usual safety precautions such as installing an entry-proof fence around your pool. The controversy about infant swimming lessons is justified. Infants may get sick from swallowing too much heavily chlorinated water. Also, we feel that the forced-dunking methods advocated by some instructors may instill a fear of swimming in the impressionable infant. Here are some suggestions on teaching your baby to swim: Be sure the water is warm, around 80°. Enroll in baby swim class which teaches *you* how to teach your baby. We have found the best results are when babies are taught along with the parents, or even better, the parent is taught how to teach the baby. Your local YMCA may offer parent–baby swim classes.

First of all, it is important for your baby to enjoy water and be in the arms of a trusted and familiar care giver. When you get into the water, hold your infant firmly in your arms with his head at the same level as your head. Lower yourself until your shoulders are submerged. The water level should be at about the baby's chest. His face should never be lower than yours because you won't be able to watch his reactions to know when to continue or when to stop. When he seems relaxed and happy, proceed to the next step—blowing bubbles. Hold your baby upright and facing you. Blow slightly against his face, then lower your mouth into the water so that he can see the bubbles you make. Let his hand feel the bubbles, and then let him copy your bubble blowing. Practice this play time and bubble blowing frequently. Going into the water six times a day for ten minutes is much better than going in once for sixty minutes. Remember to have fun. No infant or child can learn when he is unhappy. A happy, confident child is less likely to panic in a difficult situation. Retreat at the first sign of tension. Remember that you want your baby first to enjoy water; swimming is a much later step.

216. *Our two-year-old is very curious, and I am afraid she's going to get into products in our medicine cabinet. What precautions should we take?*

Try the following accident-prevention tips:

1. Be certain all medicines and potentially harmful substances are packaged in safety containers. Leave the safety cap on when you are using the substance.
2. Put safety latches on cupboards and medicine cabinets.
3. Store potentially harmful chemicals such as insecticides and petroleum products in a safe place beyond the reach of your child.
4. Avoid referring to medicine as candy.
5. Keep an emetic (a substance which induces vomiting) in your home medicine kit. We recommend syrup of Ipecac. To induce vomiting give your child one tablespoon (15 cc's) of Ipecac in eight ounces of water or noncarbonated fruit juice. Jostling or bouncing your baby on your knee may hasten the vomiting. If vomiting does not occur within twenty minutes, give one more tablespoon of Ipecac in juice or water. Perform this ritual in the bathroom or kitchen. Often it is unnecessary to induce vomiting if the substance is not toxic or the dosage small.

    Do not induce vomiting for the following products: (1) cleaning fluids such as bleach and ammonia; (2) petroleum products including gasoline, kerosene, benzene, and turpentine; (3) strong corrosives such as lye, strong acids and drain cleaners; (4) polishes including furniture and car polish. Before inducing vomiting, always check with your local poison-control center. Consult your local hospital or the yellow pages to find the nearest poison-control center, and display the phone number in a conspicuous place. Most poison-control centers have stickers with their phone number. Ask for these stickers and place them on your phones.

217. *Our toddler likes to chew on furniture and his crib bars. Can he get lead poisoning from this?*

In the mid-seventies laws limited the content of lead in house paint and in paint used on children's toys and furniture. If the furniture has been made and painted within the last fifteen years, it is unlikely that the paint contains enough lead to harm your child. The paint on imported furniture, however, may not be subject to as stringent lead-content laws as domestic furniture, so you have to be more careful with this furniture. Older baby furniture, such as cribs, may contain paint with very high lead content, which can be toxic to your child. If this is the case, strip the baby furniture of the old paint and repaint using a newer non-lead paint. Be careful of purchasing repainted secondhand furniture, since the old paint underneath may be high in lead. Keep your little beaver from chewing on older painted wood. Newer cribs have plastic strips on the top of the crib bars to discourage chewing on the wood.

218. *I've heard that aspirin may not be safe for babies. Is this true? When can I safely use aspirin and when should I not?*

Aspirin is generally being replaced by acetaminophen in pediatrics today, primarily because of the controversy surrounding the possible association between aspirin and Reye's syndrome—a potentially fatal disease. Researchers are divided as to whether a cause and effect or a coincidental relationship exists between Reye's syndrome and the use of aspirin in certain conditions such as chicken pox and flu. Until this question is answered, pediatricians recommend not using aspirin for chicken pox or the flu. Acetaminophen is safer than aspirin and equally as effective in lowering fever. Acetaminophen has the following advantages:

1. It has not been implicated as a cause of Reye's syndrome.
2. It is available in tablet and liquid form, and is therefore easier to administer to young children.
3. Your child is less likely to get sick from an overdose of acetaminophen than with aspirin. Acetaminophen has a wider range between the dosage that is needed to be effective and the dosage that is toxic to your child.

Aspirin, however, is more effective than acetaminophen

in relieving muscle and joint aches. Therefore, your doctor may suggest its use for this purpose. In general, use acetaminophen instead of aspirin to control your child's fever. If you must use aspirin, administer only the recommended dose and do not give aspirin to your child longer than forty-eight hours without rechecking with your doctor.

219. *Our two-year-old is always putting things into her mouth, and I'm worried that she will swallow things such as pennies. How will I know whether these are harmful to her? What do I do if she chokes?*

Children occasionally do swallow small objects such as coins. These nearly always pass through the intestines and are eliminated in twenty-four to forty-eight hours without causing any harm. Rarely do swallowed objects obstruct the intestines. The main concern is if the object obstructs breathing or swallowing. Here are some worry signs: difficulty swallowing, excessive drooling, excessive abdominal pain, or any signs of difficulty breathing. Sometimes an object such as a rock may lodge in a child's esophagus, the tube running from the mouth to the stomach. Pain in the area where the object is stuck plus excessive drooling are signs of this type of obstruction. If your child exhibits no signs that the swallowed object is bothering her, the object will probably pass without harm. X rays are rarely necessary to confirm the presence or absence of a coin if your child is not showing any of the symptoms listed above. Just wait a day or two and you'll get your money back!

If your child starts choking, observe the following steps:

1. If she can speak, cry, and cough, the airway is not completely obstructed and you should not interfere with her own efforts to dislodge the material. If she is not panicky and is breathing normally, give her emotional support and allow her own cough reflex to dislodge the object.
2. If she is having difficulty getting air, is blue, or is losing consciousness, place her head down over your lap or

along your arm and administer four hard, quick back blows with the palm of your hand between the shoulder blades. Repeat if necessary. The back blow procedure is the most effective in the choking child. The Heimlich maneuver is generally not recommended for infants and small children because of the danger of damage to the abdominal organs.

3. Unless you can see the object and are certain you can get your finger around it, do not use your finger to dislodge foreign bodies from the back of a child's throat. Doing so may push the object farther back into the child's small throat, or may cause her to panic and suck the object into the lungs rather than swallow it.

All parents should take a CPR course such as one offered by your local Red Cross. In these courses you will learn safe methods for treating the choking child. (See Appendix for suggested CPR resources.)

220. *Our one-year-old often runs a high temperature when ill. I don't like giving him medicines all the time just for the fever. I've also heard that fever will help a child fight an infection. Is this true?*

Yes. There is a scant bit of research which suggests that an elevated body temperature may help the body's normal defense mechanisms fight an infection. It is not necessary to treat a low fever (100–101°F. rectally). With higher temperatures (102–104°F.), this theoretical evidence gives way to practical considerations. A high fever makes a child very uncomfortable, so you may want to give him medicine to lessen the discomfort. Watch your child during a febrile illness. When the temperature is high, he will probably just lie around, moan, and seem generally uncomfortable (although being quiet is actually beneficial). As soon as the fever breaks, the previously hot child will be up and playing and obviously feeling better. If the temperature goes too high too quickly, a convulsion may occur. The immature brain of the infant and young child is particularly prone to convulsions if the fever shoots up too quickly. That is the main reason to control a child's fever with medicine.

Turn down the temperature in your child's room, thus keeping his environment cool. Allow circulation of air by opening a window slightly or by using an air conditioner or nearby fan. A draft will not make your child sick.

If your child's temperature is over 103°F. (39.5°C.) or he seems to be very uncomfortable, you can often lower his temperature by placing him in a tepid bath. Sit him in approximately twelve inches of tepid bath water and sit in the tub with him. Play with your child and keep him quiet. Rub his body with washcloths while he is in the tub. This action stimulates blood circulation to his skin, allowing the heat to come out into the cooler water. A twenty-minute tub bath usually brings the temperature down at least one or two degrees. Do not use alcohol rubs to lower temperature. The vapor may irritate the child's lungs. After the bath, pat him dry with a towel, leaving a slight amount of water on his skin. This will evaporate and cool him more. If you have given him the proper dose of medication to reset his thermostat as we have mentioned above, he will not shiver during this bath and cooling procedure.

221. *Our eighteen-month-old is prone to convulsions whenever she has a fever. What is the best way to control fever?*

Using the analogy of temperature control in your house may help you understand your child's body temperature. If your house is too warm, you lower the thermostat and open the windows. If you open the windows but do not reset the thermostat, the furnace increases the heat production and your house remains warm. The same goes for treating fever in your child. You must, in effect, reset the thermostat and "open the windows." Here's how: First, give your child an appropriate dosage of acetaminophen or aspirin; these temperature-lowering medicines reset her body thermostat so that she will not produce more heat. Next, lower the temperature in her environment to allow heat to get out.

This is one aspect of child care where a mother's intuition seems to fail. Mothers often intuitively want to bundle their child up with extra clothing during a fever. Do exactly the opposite. Undress your child completely or dress her in light, loose-fitting garments. This allows her body heat to radiate into the much cooler environment.

222. *I am confused about how to take our baby's temperature. Can you give me some guidelines?*

Take his temperature after he has been quiet for a half hour. A screaming baby or a child who has been running around may show a temperature one or two degrees higher than when quiet. Practice feeling your child's temperature by placing the palm of your hand on his forehead or by kissing his forehead so that you can tell when his temperature is normal and when it is elevated. If your touch suggests that your child has a fever, confirm this by taking his temperature with a thermometer. Buy one which is easiest for you to read. Some are easier than others. You can buy digital thermometers which give you a number reading. You can take your child's temperature in three places: the rectum, armpit, or mouth. Rectal temperature is one half to one degree higher than oral temperature, and axillary temperature is usually one degree lower than oral. Shake down the thermometer with a wrist-snapping motion until the mercury column is below 95°F. Hold the thermometer tightly as you shake it, or do it over a bed or soft surface in case you drop it. A rectal thermometer is the easiest and most accurate device to use for babies. The only difference between oral and rectal thermometers is in the tip. The rectal thermometer is short and stubby to prevent injury to the rectal tissue. The tip of the oral thermometer is long and thin. To take your child's rectal temperature, follow these steps:

1. Shake down the thermometer. Grease the bulb end with petroleum jelly.

2. Lay your child facedown across your lap.
3. Gently insert the thermometer bulb about one inch into the rectum. Allow the thermometer to seek its own path. Don't force it.
4. Hold the thermometer in place between your index and middle fingers with the palm of your hand and your fingers grasping your baby's buttocks. This way you can hold the thermometer and keep him from moving. Never leave a baby alone with a thermometer in place.
5. Try to keep the thermometer in place for three minutes. If your child is struggling, one minute may be long enough to give a reading within a degree of the true temperature.

To take your baby's axillary temperature you can use either a rectal or oral thermometer. Follow these steps:

1. Have your baby sit on your lap and hold him firmly with one arm around his shoulder.
2. Wipe his armpit dry. Lift his arm and gently place the bulb of the thermometer into the armpit. Hold his arm flat against his chest, closing the armpit.
3. Allow at least three minutes to get an accurate axillary temperature; five minutes is better.

During your baby's next checkup, ask your doctor's nurse to show you how to take your baby's temperature.

223. *My baby has thrush. Is this serious and what can I do about it?*

Thrush is a common fungus infection of the mouth. It looks like white patches on your baby's inner cheeks, tongue and roof of the mouth. Thrush seldom bothers or causes a baby problems and is easily treated by applying prescription medication. Sometimes a fungus diaper rash occurs along with oral thrush, and a prescription cream may be necessary. If your baby has thrush and you are breastfeeding, the thrush may occasionally be transmitted to your nipples. Applying some of your baby's oral thrush medicine to your nipples will prevent this. Usually oral thrush will disappear after a week of medication; sometimes thrush may persist and need several weeks of treatment.

224. *Several children in my daughter's preschool have developed head lice and now she has them too. I feel terribly embarrassed because I do keep our house clean. What can I do?*

First of all, don't feel embarrassed. The fact that your daughter has head lice is not a reflection on the cleanliness of your home, your economic status, or personal hygiene. Head lice are everywhere that there are a lot of children in small spaces such as classrooms. Head lice do not fly or jump but are transmitted by direct contact, such as by sharing grooming aids like combs and brushes and by sharing caps and scarfs. Teach your child not to share these personal items.

Head lice are too tiny to be seen with the naked eye. You need a magnifying glass to spot them. You're most likely to see the nits (the eggs), which look like tiny specks of sugar, adhering to the base of the hair shaft near the nape of the neck or around the ears. If you see these nits, don't panic; they are easy to eliminate. Treatment of head lice is much easier nowadays than it used to be. The newer over-the-counter shampoos are almost as effective and much safer than the stronger prescription shampoos of yesteryear. These shampoos come with a specially designed nit comb which removes the nits without damaging the hair shaft. Shampoo your child's hair as directed and repeat the shampooing seven to ten days later. Thoroughly wash personal articles such as combs, brushes, scarves, hats, towels and bed clothing—anything which touches the hair—in very hot water. Dry clothing and linens in the hot cycle in the dryer, or have the items dry-cleaned. If this is impractical, placing items in a sealed plastic bag for ten days will kill the lice and eggs. If your child has head lice, don't treat her like a leper. They are not highly contagious, and are more a source of discomfort and embarrassment than a real medical problem.

225. *Our two-year-old has a cold that has lingered on for two weeks. Our doctor checked him last week and didn't find anything wrong, but now he seems to be getting worse. Should I consult another doctor?*

Not necessarily. When your doctor initially examined your child, he may have simply had a cold. Most colds go away without medication. Sometimes, however, a cold progresses into a chest or ear infection and gets worse if untreated. Thus doctors always advise parents to check back with them if the cold has gotten worse. Notify your doctor that your child's cold has become more severe and that you would like him to be checked again. It is often necessary for a doctor to change his diagnosis if the condition of the child changes.

226. *Our two-year-old coughs a lot and I'm worried about pneumonia. How can I tell if she's contacted this infection?*

Parents and grandparents often worry about pneumonia, perhaps because of memories from years ago when it was a serious illness. With modern antibiotics, pneumonia is not as serious as it used to be. Many doctors now use the term *chest infection* rather than pneumonia so as not to alarm grandparents. There are two types of pneumonia: the old-fashioned type, with a high fever, chills, severe cough, and a very sick-looking child. This type of pneumonia usually gets better within a few days after treatment with antibiotics. The other type of pneumonia, also called walking pneumonia, is a more lingering type of lung infection in which the child is not particularly sick, but may take longer to get better. These two types of infections result from different types of germs, which cause different symptoms and require different types of treatment. With most cases of pneumonia your doctor can hear the infection by listening to your child's chest; she can then prescribe accordingly. Sometimes a chest

X ray is necessary to confirm the diagnosis. Remember, don't tell grandmother that your child has pneumonia; she has a "chest infection."

227. *Our three-year-old often gets throat infections. I've heard pediatricians are hesitant to take tonsils out as much as they used to a generation ago. Is this true?*

Yes and no. Fewer tonsillectomies are performed today, but it is still a widely used and often a necessary operation. Following are the usual reasons for removing your child's tonsils:

1. Tonsil infections are becoming more frequent, more severe, and are increasingly accompanied by ear infections.
2. The tonsils are enlarging, causing obstruction to breathing and swallowing, often evident from the child's loud snoring at night.
3. The number of doctor's visits and school absences are increasing steadily, due to tonsil infections.

   If any of these criteria are present, then your child may need his tonsils and/or adenoids removed. Often the tonsils increase in size until around four years of age; thereafter, they begin to shrink and the number of tonsil infections diminishes. The doctor who knows your child the best is the one who should make the decision about tonsillectomy.

228. *Our three-month-old infant is formula fed and gets constipated frequently. She is very uncomfortable when this occurs. What can I do to relieve her constipation?*

Try the following remedies: Some formulas produce more constipation than others, so experiment with various formulas to determine which one causes the softest stool. If your baby strains with each bowel movement, give a glycerine suppository every other day for a week or two. These look like small bullets and are available without prescription at your local pharmacy. Give your baby around eight ounces of additional water each day, especially during the warmer seasons. Stool softeners added to her formula are usually not necessary at this age but may be prescribed by your physician if the above measures do not work. Since your baby is prone to constipation, it would be wise to delay the introduction of constipation-producing solids such as rice and bananas.

229. *Our three-year-old is chronically constipated. Even when he does have a bowel movement, it's only a small amount. He soils his pants frequently. How can we help him?*

Constipation is one of the most uncomfortable and perplexing problems in the young child. This is how the system is normally designed to work: The presence of a lot of stool in the large intestine signals an urge to defecate. The child either responds to this signal or chooses to ignore it if he is too busy playing. Unlike the urge to urinate, which a child usually cannot control for long, he can choose to ignore his signal to defecate. The longer he ignores it, the more the fluid in the retained stool is absorbed and the harder the stools become. It then hurts to go to the bathroom, causing the child to hold on to his stools even longer, and the vicious cycle begins—he holds on to his stool longer and longer and becomes more and more constipated. Sometimes intestinal fluid may leak out around the hard stool, resulting in soiling of the child's pants. Parents may even regard frequent pants soiling as diarrhea when it is really a by-product of constipation.

Try the following with your child: Make a diagram of the large intestine, showing large "golf balls" of stool at the end of the large intestine. Show your child that voluntarily holding on to his stools make them harder and that is why it hurts to pass them. Also show him how the fluid leaks around the stool, causing the embarrassing soiled pants. Encourage him to have a bowel movement at set times during the day, mainly after breakfast. Encourage him to respond to his urge to go promptly. Convey to him that he should "go when you have to go."

If your child has had this problem for a long time, the intestinal muscles may be somewhat weakened and a month of stool softening may be needed before this problem is corrected. Begin with natural laxatives such as prunes and prune juice, bran flakes, psyllium husks (similar to bran flakes but more effective). The following foods also act as laxatives: fruit, prune juice, corn syrup, vegetable roughage and bran cereal. Potentially constipating foods are: rice, cheese, bananas, chocolate, and sometimes milk; these foods should not be eaten in large quantities. Consult your physician about the use of laxatives which are stool softeners, such as mineral oil. If the constipation is severe, you may have to start with a clean slate by giving your child an enema.

230. *Our three-year-old complains of stomach aches frequently. Our doctor has thoroughly examined her and tells us not to worry. When should we be concerned?*

You have gone through the first important step—taking your child to the doctor for a thorough examination. It sounds as if your doctor has reassured you that, at least for the moment, there is nothing going on in your child that will eventually cause harm if left untreated. Many children have vague abdominal pains throughout early and middle childhood. A cause is seldom found for these pains, and many of them eventually disappear. I would suggest that you keep a diary and accurately record the events surrounding these pains: the dates they occur, the time of the day, the events just before the onset of the pain, what makes it get worse, what makes it get better, etc. Try to identify the trigger. Are these pains related to meals? type of food? type of activity? stress? time of day? If your child is consistently vague in the description of the pains, if they follow no consistent pattern or association with events or food, and if they are not increasing in severity or frequency, you do not have to worry. Another sign of when to worry is whether or not these pains occur at night. In general, any pain that awakens the child from sleep is of much more concern than those when she is awake. If these abdominal pains do not awaken your child, they are less of a worry.

Constipation and food allergies are the most common causes of abdominal pain at three years of age. Be sure your child is not constipated. If she is, discuss with your doctor the use of laxatives and a change of diet. Keep a list of foods that your child has eaten and see if you can determine a relationship between these foods and subsequent pains. The usual culprits, in order of frequency, are: dairy products, wheat, eggs, soy, nuts, corn, chocolate, and berries. Any foods in excess may also cause abdominal pain. You may try an elimination diet, requiring your child to avoid each one of these foods for a period of two to three weeks. If you notice a change, reintroduce the suspected food to see if the pain recurs.

Observe the "one-finger sign" when diagnosing abdominal pain. Ask your child to point to where it hurts. If she uses her whole hand to encircle her abdomen in the general location of the navel, but cannot pinpoint the exact site of the pain, this is less of a worry. If, however, she puts one finger on the site of the pain, this is of more concern. Keep in close contact with your doctor if the pains change in character, increase in frequency and severity, or seem to be accompanied by signs that your child is generally unwell.

231. *Our newborn's feet and legs curve in markedly. Will this correct itself?*

Yes. Newborns have bowed legs and in-turned feet because of the position that they lay in the womb. Because no "standing room" exists in your womb, your baby naturally draws his legs up over his abdomen and curves his feet inward. This position causes the leg bones to be twisted inward, resulting in the combination of bowed legs and in-turned feet. These curvatures nearly always correct themselves. During the first year your pediatrician will check your baby's leg growth to make sure these curvatures are straightening out normally. You can help your baby's feet and legs straighten out by discouraging sleep in the fetal position. Babies like to sleep on their tummies with their feet and legs curled up underneath them as they did in the womb. By repeatedly pulling his feet out from under him while sleeping, you will help your baby stop this habit.

In addition to these normal, self-correcting bone curvatures, one or both feet may be turned in because the front of the foot is curved inward in relation to the back of the foot, a condition called forefoot adduction. Your doctor will discuss this type of foot problem on your baby's first checkup. If, without a great deal of force, you can stretch the front of the foot in line with the back of the foot, only a minor problem exists. This problem is easily treated by periodic stretching exercises which your doctor will demonstrate to you. If you stroke the skin on the outside of your infant's foot and he voluntarily straightens his foot, no deformity exists and no treatment is necessary. If his foot is not straightening out normally during the first few months, your doctor may recommend orthopedic treatment.

232. *Our fifteen-month-old toes-in a lot when she walks. She walks well and doesn't trip often, but her gait looks awkward. Will this correct itself?*

Yes, usually. Most toddlers who toe-in (pigeon-toed) have normal feet and legs. Most toeing-in is the result of inward curvature of the lower leg bones (called internal tibial torsion). The feet simply follow the leg. Most toeing-in problems correct themselves by two or three years of age. Another reason why toddlers normally toe-in is to compensate for flat feet. Most children do not develop much of an arch until three to four years of age. Between two or three years of age a child toes-in to compensate for an absent arch by shifting the weight to the outside of the foot. As the arch develops, the toeing-in lessens.

As a general rule, you should not worry if your child's toeing-in does not cause her to trip over her feet while walking or running. Keep a diary. If she is tripping less and the toeing-in is gradually lessening as she approaches two to two and a half, treatment is seldom necessary. If your child is tripping more and the toeing-in is not correcting itself, orthopedic treatment may be necessary even between eighteen months and two years of age. One simple treatment you can try is to discourage your child from sleeping in the fetal position with her legs curled up underneath her. Sneak in while she is sleeping and pull her legs out from underneath her during naps and after she goes to sleep at night.

233. *Our two-year-old has knock-knees. It doesn't bother him, but it looks unusual. What can we do?*

Between the ages of two and six years, nearly all children show some degree of knock-knees. This is due to the laxity of the ligaments supporting the inside of the knee joint. When your child stands, the ligaments supporting the inside of the knees stretch easily, allowing the knees to cave inward. This appearance is aggravated by the ligament laxity around the ankle joint, allowing the ankles to curve outward. As your child grows, the ligaments supporting the inside of the knees and ankles strengthen and the knees knock less. You can help your child correct this knock-kneed appearance by teaching him to sit Indian style or in the tailor position (feet turned toward each other in front of child) and not with his legs turned outward when he sits on the floor (a position called the W position). This position stretches the inner ligaments of the knees and ankles, aggravating the already caved-in appearance of the toddler with knock-knees and out-turned ankles.

234. *Our one-year-old toes out a lot, causing her to walk peculiarly. Will this correct itself?*

Yes. Most toddlers voluntarily turn their feet out when they are beginning to walk. This seems to increase their balance much in the same way a ballerina stands with her feet turned out for balance. Turning out is seldom due to an orthopedic problem and usually corrects itself as your toddler improves her balance during walking.

235. *Our two-year-old has very flat feet. So does his father. Should we worry about this? And what can be done?*

Flat feet are often due to heredity. Some infants inherit stretchy ligaments which cause their ankles to turn out, giving the appearance of flat feet. The foot itself is normally flat throughout infancy. Young infants have "fat pads" which obscure the arch of the foot. As the infant grows, this fat pad disappears and reveals an arch around two years of age. When your child stands, the previously visible arch may disappear and the feet may again appear flat. This is because the ligaments that normally bind the bones and the arch together cannot support the weight on these bones and so the arch appears to collapse. As your child grows, these ligaments strengthen enough to support his weight. The child may exhibit an arch by the age of three or four. Between two and four years of age, if his flat feet are not disturbing his walking, you need not worry. The choice of treatment of your child's flat feet depends on whether there is undue strain on the ligaments of the foot. The easiest way to detect this is to look at your child's heel from behind. If the ankle tendon is perpendicular to the floor, his axis of weight bearing is normal and no abnormal stress is placed on the flat foot. If his heel is slanted outward, unnecessary strain is placed upon the foot. If left untreated, this strain may result in leg pains, aggravation of knock-knees, and persistent out-turned heels and sore feet in later childhood. If your child exhibits this out-turned-heel appearance, one of the most effective treatments is to place custom-molded plastic inserts, called orthotics, inside regular shoes. Orthopedists usually recommend orthotics around the age of four.

236. *Our nine-month-old baby is pulling herself up on the furniture and trying to stand. When should I consider buying her first pair of shoes?*

Foot specialists are divided on when babies should wear their first pair of shoes. Some feel that babies should learn to walk barefoot. After she has been walking for a couple of months, you may try some shoes. Your baby's feet will develop just as well without any type of footwear, but most parents find that shoes are necessary for the beginning walker. Shoes help protect your baby's tender feet from the rough surfaces, splinters, and sharp objects that lie in her path. When she is learning to walk, she looks ahead, not down, and these uncautious little feet are likely to bump into anything.

Some foot specialists feel that shoes help a baby walk better, others do not. The reason why shoes may help some babies walk better is that the flat, even bottoms of the shoes provide lateral stability for a young tenderfoot. Walking is a balancing act. Your baby balances on one foot while swinging the other foot ahead. Shoes on a baby's feet are like flippers on a scuba diver—they square off and widen the margins of the foot, providing a steady, stable surface for the balancing foot while the free foot forges ahead. The insole of the shoe also provides a surface for your baby's toes to first grip and then push off of when taking a step. If the walking surface is soft and yielding, such as a thick, carpet or a sponge pad in a playpen, a barefoot baby's toes may sink in too much and make walking difficult. When your baby is beginning to take her first steps, you may try having her fitted for her first pair of shoes. If she walks better in them, she is ready. (See question 237 on selecting a baby's footwear.) If she trips a lot, she is not.

237. *What should we look for in a good pair of shoes for our baby, who is just beginning to walk?*

Remember, babies' feet and walking styles are as individual as their faces and smiles. When your baby begins to take those first steps, the time for shoes has arrived. There are four parts of a shoe that you should examine:

1. **The sole.** As a general rule, the earlier the stage of walking, the thinner and more flexible the sole should be. Before buying a shoe, bend it in your hand to test its flexibility. Then watch your baby walk. The shoes should bend at the ball of the foot as he takes each step.
2. **The counter (back of the shoe).** To insure a proper fit, the counter should be firm. Try this test: Squeeze the counter between your thumb and forefinger. If it feels too soft, it will weaken with wear, causing the shoe to slip off.
3. **The heel.** With your baby's first shoe, a slight heel is advisable to help prevent dangerous backward falls.
4. **Top and side of the shoe.** Both parts should crease easily when your baby takes a step. If they don't, it means his shoe is not flexible enough and the foot can't bend naturally while walking.

Selecting an experienced shoe salesperson is one of the most important steps in caring for your baby's feet. When you try on shoes yourself, you can usually tell whether they fit by the way they feel. But your baby cannot tell you whether a particular shoe feels right or not. So, just as you trust your pediatrician to advise you properly through your baby's developmental stages, you should be able to trust your shoe fitter for advice on your baby's footwear needs. A well-trained salesperson understands and practices progression fitting. This means properly matching the changes in shoe size and design with the progressive changes in a child's style of walking and foot development.

Parents often ask about high-top shoes. Since a baby's heel is not well defined for at least the first two years, there is little to hold the foot in the shoe. This is why some babies need higher shoes than others, depending on the development of the heel. Many babies do well in a three-quarter boot, which is not as high as the traditional high-top and gives the ankle more freedom of movement while

staying on your baby's foot just as well. A well-trained shoe
salesperson can advise you as to what height of shoe is best
for your baby.

238. *Do I need to spend a lot of money on our baby's
shoes, or are inexpensive sneakers all right?*

The most common problem with cheap shoes is fit. Studies
have shown that only one in every four babies have so-called
average feet and can get a good fit with inexpensive shoes,
which may come only in medium widths and full sizes. The
great majority of toddlers have either short, pudgy feet or
long, narrow ones or some other odd but lovable shape that
makes them unique. To meet the special fitting needs of
most babies, quality shoes are made in a wide variety of
widths and in both full and half sizes. However, the higher
quality of the material in the shoe and the necessity of
keeping such a large inventory of sizes adds to the cost of
babies shoes.

Leather soles are generally superior to rubber soles
because they are much more flexible. Leather becomes more
flexible with increasing wear and gradually conforms to the
shape of the foot. Thick rubber soles, like those found on
some inexpensive sneakers, are usually too stiff and may
catch on certain surfaces, causing a nasty fall. I have seen
many parents incur medical bills for repair of a laceration
to their infant's forehead after she tripped due to improperly
fitting shoes. Recent studies conducted at Stanford University and the University of Vermont show that rubber-soled
sneakers are less flexible than leather-soled shoes and that
toddlers stumble and fall more in sneakers than in leather
shoes. Two-year-olds wearing sneakers in the Vermont study
had an awkward plop-plop gait, lifting one leg and placing
it in front of the other. The same children wearing leather
shoes fell less often and walked more naturally.

Most sneakers are made of canvas or nylon. Better-
quality baby shoes are made of leather. Since leather is a
natural skin, it allows your baby's foot to breathe. As a

result, feet stay dryer and more comfortable in leather shoes. Leather also protects against extremes in temperature, keeping a baby's feet cool in summer and warm in winter. Because canvas does not have the same breathing qualities as leather, heat and perspiration are trapped inside your baby's shoes and her feet are more susceptible to rashes, athlete's foot, and other foot infections.

The sole is another advantage of leather shoes over rubber-soled sneakers. Leather soles are flat and provide more lateral stability for your baby, while many rubber-soled sneakers have rounded edges, which can encourage your baby's feet to roll inward or outward. A parent who buys a better baby shoe is also paying for the expertise of a qualified shoe fitter. A properly fitting shoe may save your baby a costly accident. (See Appendix for suggested resources on infant footwear.)

239. *How will I know when my baby needs a new pair of shoes?*

Most toddlers outgrow shoes before they outwear them. During the first year your baby is walking, she may go through three or four pairs. Since a baby's feet don't follow any consistent growth pattern, you must check her shoe size every two to three months. Here's what to check to see if your baby has outgrown her shoes:

1. Toe room. While your child is standing, you can feel her pinkie or little toe, pressing against the inside of her shoe.
2. Throat room (area across the top of the shoe just below the laces). The leather across the throat looks very tight and there is no give when you pinch it.
3. The counter. The back of the shoe hangs over the heel either on the inner side or outer side of the shoe.

Also, be sure to examine your baby's feet each time you remove her shoes. If her toes are curled or you notice marks or indentations in the skin, her shoes are almost certainly too tight.

240. *Our one-year-old is just beginning to walk. Is it all right to give him hand-me-down shoes from his older sister?*

In general, do not use hand-me-down shoes. The size of babies' feet, style of walking, and weight-bearing character-istics are all different. Your older child has molded his baby shoes to conform to his own feet. This is especially true of high-quality soft leather shoes, which tend to custom mold to the individual feet and walking style.

241. *How can I get our eighteen-month-old to brush her teeth?*

It is important to brush an infant's teeth. Since yours is eighteen months, you can capitalize on two natural urges: "Just like mommy" and "All by myself." While you are brushing your teeth, encourage your toddler to watch. It is usually better to wait until she shows some interest in brushing her teeth. When she shows a desire to brush, give her her own toothbrush and show her how. Place a mirror on the bathroom wall at her level so she can watch herself brush her own teeth.

The frequency of brushing and the way you brush is more important than how long you brush your infant's teeth. Children's toothbrushes should have soft bristles and should be replaced frequently. A brush with bent bristles does not clean properly. Although I encourage you to teach your child to brush her own teeth, most children under the age of four years do not clean their own teeth effectively. If your infant refuses a toothbrush, try this: Place her on your lap face up with her feet pointing away from you. Using a 2"x2" piece of gauze wrapped around your forefinger, vigorously wipe her teeth and gums. Let your finger be her toothbrush. Some dentists recommend that you clean your baby's gums even before the teeth erupt.

Certain circumstances require extra dental care. If your child uses a nighttime bottle, try to use only water. Sugary beverages such as juice or even milk increase your child's risk of dental caries because the natural rinsing action of saliva is diminished during sleep. If she insists on milk or juice, brush her teeth afterward or at least the next morning. This is important if your baby nurses a lot at night. After your child eats sticky foods such as raisins, dates, and prunes, brush her teeth. Even though she will eventually lose all of her baby teeth, these primary teeth serve as spacers to encourage proper alignment of the permanent teeth. These little teeth are valuable; take good care of them.

Forced teeth brushing in a reluctant child may create a negative attitude toward dental hygiene. Early gum cleaning helps condition a younger baby to expect and cooperate with oral hygiene. Once your child is verbal enough to understand, it helps to explain *why* teeth must be brushed. We used the concept of "sugar bugs" to get our two-and-a-half-year-old to be excited about brushing—he took great delight in attacking those "sugar bugs" with his toothbrush and then letting me check to make sure he got them all.

242. *We have a hard time brushing our two-year-old's teeth. Any suggestions?*

It is necessary to brush a child's teeth at least twice a day. Rarely can a two-year-old brush his own teeth effectively, so you must do it for him. Try the following: Show him that teeth brushing is fun. Let him sit next to the washbasin and watch you brush your teeth. Hand him his own toothbrush and let him mirror your tooth brushing while you sing a song or play a teeth-brushing game such as "Let's brush our teeth together to get the sugar bugs off." Use a toothbrush with soft bristles and run it under hot water to further soften them. Hard bristles on tender gums discourage the reluctant tooth brusher. If your child resists the use of a toothbrush, wrap a piece of gauze around your index finger and use your finger as a brush. Use a children's toothpaste which has a milder flavor and a favorite cartoon character on the package. As with so many aspects of child rearing, brushing a child's teeth is half good hygiene and half creative marketing.

243. *Our family tree is littered with relatives with dental problems. What can I do to help our baby have good teeth?*

The following is a list of dental-care tips that we have found increase the chances of a child having healthy teeth:

1. Breastfeed as long as possible.
2. Use fluoride supplements in areas which do not have adequate fluoride in the water.
3. Begin brushing your baby's teeth and gums at least by one year of age.
4. Avoid nighttime bottles or milk or juice. If the baby breastfeeds at night, clean her teeth first thing in the morning.
5. Avoid plaque foods. Plaque is an invisible sticky film that is constantly forming on the teeth and contains harmful bacteria. This bacteria acts on the sugar in food and forms a decay-producing acid, which is held against the teeth by the plaque. Avoid those foods which cause prolonged contact of sugar on the teeth, such as lollipops and hard candy, which can lodge upon and between the teeth. Many sticky foods are healthy, such as raisins, dates, and prunes, but they need to be brushed off your child's teeth after feeding.
6. Observe regular dental checkups after the age of two years.

244. *Our six-month-old baby seems to be in pain while he is cutting teeth. How can I help him?*

"Cutting" teeth is exactly what happens. At birth your baby's teeth are inside the gum. Around six months (the time of teething varies widely, anywhere between four and eight months or even later) the baby teeth begin to cut through the edge of the gum. Naturally this causes pressure and pain on the gums and bothers many babies. The common discomforts associated with teething are a low-grade fever (seldom greater than 101°F. rectally), wakefulness, irritability, diminished appetite, increased finger sucking and gum rubbing, loose stools with a consequent diaper rash, and excessive drooling with a resulting "drool rash" on your baby's cheeks. Teething may sometimes be confused with a cold. When the drool collects in the back of his throat, your baby may cough and there may be a raspy sound to his breathing. A runny nose or watery eyes, especially if the discharge is thick and yellow, should *not* be attributed to teething.

If several teeth are erupting at the same time, babies are often extremely uncomfortable. Try the following comforting measures: acetaminophen, a cool teether such as a frozen banana, cool spoon, an ice cube in a baby sock, or massaging the gums with your finger often helps. In our experience, topical anesthetic applied to sore gums is usually ineffective. Every once in a while, slight bleeding may accompany teething of the side molars as they cut through the gums. A juice "Popsicle" or ice cube will stop the bleeding.

245. *Our baby is two years old. When should she see a dentist?*

The American Academy of Pediatrics recommends regular dental checkups beginning at age one to two years. You should certainly take your baby to a dentist for her first dental checkup when her teeth are completely in, usually by two and a half years of age. If there is a family history of dental problems or your doctor is concerned about dental abnormalities, an earlier exam may be necessary. During your baby's first dental checkup, you may ask or your doctor will cover the following important points of dental hygiene: fluoride supplements, flossing and brushing, nighttime bottles and/or nursing, and nutrition. Choose a dentist who understands that a small child needs to have a parent with her for exams and treatments. Schedule the first checkup hopefully *before* there's a problem, just so the dentist can "count" your baby's teeth and the checkup can be a fun experience without any trauma.

246. *Our ten-month-old seems to be developing yellow skin, but his eyes are not yellow. Should I worry?*

This is a common and normal condition called carotenemia. It is usually caused by eating a lot of yellow vegetables such as carrots and squash. The yellow pigment from these vegetables is deposited in the skin. This condition causes your baby no harm and will subside if he eats slightly less yellow vegetables. Eventually his system will learn to handle this yellow pigment and this condition will not occur when he gets older. This is not the same as yellow jaundice. Jaundice is characterized by yellow skin *and* yellow eyes due to the buildup of yellow bilirubin pigment in the skin. This condition usually reflects a liver or blood problem. Your doctor can reassure you about your child's yellow skin.

247. *I've heard so much controversy about immunizations that I am afraid to have my baby immunized. What should I do?*

Immunize your baby. Because of the flurry of articles concerning the possible reactions to immunizations, parents have become anxious about immunizing their children. You are in a dilemma. You will worry if you don't immunize your child and you will worry if you do. Here is some information which may help you to resolve this question in your own mind: Every vaccine, and every medicine for that matter, has what is called a benefit–risk ratio, meaning that the benefit of the vaccine must outweigh the risk. There are eight vaccines that are currently available for children: tetanus, polio, whooping cough, diphtheria, measles, mumps,

German measles, and a new HIB (or meningitis) vaccine. In all of these the benefits derived from the vaccine far outweigh the risk of an adverse reaction. In only one of these vaccines, the whooping cough, or pertussis (the P of the DPT vaccine), has there been enough adverse reactions to cause concern. In countries such as Great Britain that once stopped using this vaccine outbreaks of whooping cough became prevalent, causing them to return to routine vaccine usage.

Another consideration is the area in which you live. If you live in what are called high-risk areas—border states and states with high immigrant populations (New York, Florida, California, Texas, for example) full immunization is definitely advised. The recent concern about the whooping cough vaccine has indeed stimulated manufacturers to work on a safer yet equally effective vaccine which hopefully will be available in the near future. In the meantime, we advise you to discuss your dilemma with your doctor and to consider following the recommendations of the immunization schedule set by the American Academy of Pediatrics.

248. *We are taking an airplane flight and our six-month-old infant has had a history of ear infections. Will the high altitude bother her ears?*

Possibly yes, but here are some suggestions to minimize ear pain when flying. During takeoff and landing, breastfeed or bottle-feed your baby until the plane has reached full altitude or has completely landed. Do the same while driving up and down mountains (with both of you still buckled in your seat belts). At changes in altitude, the eustachian tubes (a tiny tube connecting the middle-ear cavity with the throat to equalize pressure on both sides of the eardrum) opens and closes as the pressure changes with the changing altitude. Babies with frequent ear infections often have eustachian tubes which do not function properly and do not adjust to changing altitudes, causing intense ear pain. Allowing your baby to suck during changing altitudes causes the eustachian tube to function better. Since it may not function well during sleep, awaken your baby for the sucking exercises during takeoff and landing. Ear pain is more common during descent of the plane than during takeoff. This is the only time that I can think of that I would recommend waking a sleeping baby. The older child can drink from a cup during takeoff and landing and help her eustachian tubes function better. Here is an additional flying tip: Choose the bulkhead seat, for this seating location gives more legroom for you to stretch out in and for your baby to crawl around in.

249. *We travel often and want to put together a first-aid kit. Any suggestions?*

The following list is what we hand out to our patients.

- Absorbant cotton
- Adhesive tape—half inch and one inch
- Band-aids—various sizes
- Steri-strips (butterfly bandages)
- Cotton-tipped swabs
- Sterile gauze square—2"x2" and 4"x4", individually wrapped
- Roll of gauze bandage—two inches wide
- Tourniquet
- Flashlight and small pen light
- Tweezers and splinter forceps
- Scissors
- Thermometer
- Tongue depressors
- Measuring spoons
- Elastic bandages: Two inch and four inch
- Large cloth, 3'x3' (useful as large bandage or sling)
- Acetaminophen and children's aspirin (see question 218 for guidelines
- Syrup of ipecac (see question 216 for usage)
- Epsom salts
- Hydrogen peroxide for wound cleansing
- Petroleum jelly

- Rubbing alcohol
- Antibiotic ointment: Neosporin or Bactroban, for example
- Analgesic ear drops (Auralgan, by prescription)
- Antiseptic solution: Betadine
- Domeboro powder (soothing solution for bathing, as directed by physician)
- Cortisone cream (as directed by physician *only*)
- Calamine lotion for itching skin, poison ivy, etc.
- Cough medicine (as recommended by physician)
- Motion sickness medications—prescription Scopolamine ear patches
- Hot-water bottle
- Cold pack
- Burn cream: prescription
- Medic alert tag for allergies or illnesses
- Phone numbers—attach to kit package: your doctor's number, national poison-control hot line number

250. *I'm confused about what type of vaporizer to buy, steam or cool mist. Does it make any difference?*

Both steam and cool-mist vaporizers have their specific purposes. In general, a cool mist from the new ultrasonic type of vaporizers provides a smaller water particle, which gets down lower into your child's breathing passages. Doctors usually advise using a cool-mist vaporizer to loosen secretions low in your child's chest. In general, cool mist penetrates better into respiratory passages.

During the winter months, however, cool mist vaporizers are often impractical. My practice has been to mostly advise the use of steam vaporizers in cold weather and cool-mist vaporizers in warm weather. Central heating during cold winter months dries out the air and can further thicken the mucus in respiratory passages. A steam vaporizer can adequately heat an average-size bedroom, allowing you to turn off the central heat at night. If using steam, be sure to place the vaporizer no closer than a few feet from your child in order to avoid burns. Use vaporizers with caution if your child is allergenic. Moisture attracts mildew and other allergens and, in some allergenic children, may worsen the mucus production. For this reason, clean the vaporizer at least twice a week. If your child is allergenic, check with your doctor before using one.

251. *Our baby is six months old and we are buying his first high chair. What should we look for?*

The following tips will help you know what to look for and how to use a high chair safely:

1. The chair should have a wide base for stability.
2. Be sure the belt attaches to the frame and not the tray. *Always* use the safety belt.
3. Be sure the tray is properly secured. Children tend to push against the tray while seated or pull on the tray when climbing into the chair.
4. Be sure the chair and tray are free of sharp edges and splinters.
5. Keep the chair away from hazards such as stoves.
6. Never allow your child to stand in the chair. If he's unhappy and wants to get out, lift him out of it.

252. *Our new baby loves her infant seat, but I am worried that she will fall out. Any suggestions on using it safely?*

Falling out of an infant seat is a common accident. Do not leave your baby unattended, even when she is sitting on the changing table or on a counter top while you do something else "just for a second." By three months of age a baby can rock from side to side and build up enough torque to roll or slide right out of the seat. When babies are about five or six months old they may roll forward in the seat and topple forward or sideways. Other tips for a safe infant seat include the following:

1. The seat should have a wide, sturdy base.
2. You should use the restraining belts at all times.

3. Place the baby in the infant seat on a low, soft surface such as a carpeted floor and not on a changing table or counter top.
4. Be sure the supporting bars are fastened securely. If they pop out of the sockets, the seat will fall backward.
5. Attach non-skid tape to the underneath surface to prevent slipping.
6. Do not use the infant seat as a substitute for a car seat.

253. *Our three-year-old just got over chicken pox. It was miserable for him and the whole family. Our one-year-old will probably get it within a week or two. How can I keep him comfortable during this illness?*

Chicken pox is still one of the most common and most uncomfortable infectious diseases. Fortunately, a chicken pox vaccine is currently being tested for routine use in all children, and will probably be available for general use within a few years. Treating chicken pox involves trying to ease the itching, controlling fever, and keeping your child from scratching to prevent scars. Having treated this very itching illness in several of our children, we advise the following Sears family remedies:

First, try the following anti-itch measures: Cut your child's fingernails as short as possible. He may even have to wear mittens at night. Dress him in lightweight cotton clothing, since sweating increases itching. A cool shower often helps. Let your child soak in a warm bath. Add two cups full of baking soda and four tablespoons of cornstarch, or you can get an over-the-counter oatmeal preparation, Aveeno Bath. These solutions may also be used on a washcloth to soak and soothe skin eruptions. Our children have found "ice rubs" very itch-relieving. Place ice cubes in a paper towel and sweep across the itchy skin. This can often be done during story time to soothe the uncomfortably itching child off to sleep. Parents in our practice have reported that tea is effective in relieving itching from chicken pox in the mouth. Calamine lotion may offer some relief. Many children need

an over-the-counter or prescription antihistamine to alleviate itching and help them sleep. Sometimes a prescription
sleeping medication, such as chlorohydrate, proves effective.

To prevent scars, cut your child's fingernails short and
strongly discourage scratching, especially on the face. In our
office we prescribe a burn cream (Silvadene) to be applied
to severe pocks on the face. This enhances healing, prevents
infection, and therefore minimizes scarring. Avoid sunburn
on healing chicken pox areas. Sun damage while the skin
is trying to regain its lost pigment can cause permanent
discoloration.

254. *Our two-year-old bruises easily and I have heard that
this may be a sign of leukemia. Since there is a lot of cancer
in our family, I am worried about this bruising. Can you
explain?*

We are frequently asked this question in our office. To
alleviate your concern, nearly every toddler shows the telltale bruises of a frequent faller. There are two categories of
bruises. Those of no concern are bruises over bones such as
the shins and forearm, the usual sites of impact when a
child falls. What you should be concerned about are widespread bruises over areas that are seldom involved in physical impact such as the face and abdomen. Bruising due to
any form of cancer in a child is almost always associated
with other obvious signs of illness such as extreme paleness,
weight loss, fatigue, and physical signs (lumps, swollen
organs) that your doctor may detect on a thorough
examination.

7

BEHAVIOR PROBLEMS

The main theme of this chapter is that a child who feels right acts right. Most questions on behavior involve the subject of discipline—a term grossly misunderstood by many people. New parents often ask during their baby's eighteen-month checkup, "Should we start disciplining our baby now?" Our response is: "You began disciplining your child from the moment of birth." Children who are the products of the style of parenting we teach throughout this book—attachment parenting—are easier to discipline because as infants they feel right, and infants who feel right are more likely to act right. This inner feeling of rightness is the beginning of a baby's self-esteem. The attachment style of parenting allows a mutual trust to develop between caregiver and child. Trust is the basis of authority; a child who inwardly trusts her authority figure is easier to discipline. Discipline is an attitude that must develop within the child, forming an inner set of controls, not as an external force from outside the

225

child. In studying the children in our practice who were reared with the attachment style of parenting, we noted one common characteristic—they were easier to discipline. Why? Because these children operated from a basis of trust. In this chapter we show you how to get inside your child and understand why she acts the way she does. When you understand your child's behavior, it is easier to discipline her and channel undesirable behavior.

Admittedly, the ease with which you can discipline your child is to a great extent determined by her temperament. However, a baby who has an inner feeling of rightness seems to have a greater receptivity to being directed, as if direction, or discipline, reinforces this feeling. An inner feeling of wrongness within a child makes her less receptive of direction either from within or without herself, and accounts for the frustration of parents who state, "We just can't get through to her." We feel that the most important stage of discipline is the period from birth to one year of age. During this period you are developing sensitivity to your baby, getting to know her, maturing your intuition, and helping your baby feel right. During this time you create an attitude in your child and an atmosphere in your home that makes punishment seldom necessary, and when it is, it is administered more wisely. Throughout this book in general and in this chapter in particular, we have discussed the tools of attachment parenting and therefore the tools of discipline. We encourage a "high-touch" style of parenting, which is so necessary in this high-tech world.

255. *Our one-month-old is such a good baby. He sleeps most of the time and sometimes I even have to awaken him for feeding. Is there such a thing as a baby being too good?*

Yes. In fact, we call this the *too-good baby syndrome*. It could be that you are blessed with a baby with a very easy temperament, one of these very mellow babies that you read about or that your friends seem to have. Every baby is born with a certain temperament which corresponds to the level of need that they have in order to thrive. For example, some need to be picked up and fed often and therefore fuss if they are not picked up. Other babies are content to lie quietly in a crib and do not protest if they are not held. Usually the way the mother–infant care system works is that the infant initiates the care-giving behavior, meaning that when the baby gives you signals that he needs to be picked up, you pick him up. Some babies also need to be fed every two or three hours and fuss if their schedule is not met. Others are more content to space feedings a little longer.

Some babies, however, only seem to have lower needs, such as your baby, but may actually be high-need babies in easy-baby disguise. These infants need and enjoy being picked up and fed often, but do not have the personality to demand what they need. In other words, they do not initiate the interaction. In this case, parents need to do it, purposely carrying, holding, and feeding the baby more often than the baby actually demands.

The "too-good baby syndrome" may pose a few medical concerns. Sometimes a baby will not thrive unless he has a high level of holding, carrying, and touching. All babies grow, but not all babies thrive. Thriving implies growing to the fullest potential. The "thriving look" is the sparkly eyes, rosy cheeks, and happy appearance. If your baby seems to be thriving well, then he may not be a "too-good baby." If your doctor is not concerned about his rate of growth and development, you don't need to worry. If you or your doctor feel, however, that your baby is not thriving to his fullest potential, pick him up and hold him more often, even if he does not apparently need it.

There are rare medical conditions that may cause babies to appear too good, such as hypothyroidism. This is routinely checked at birth, and your doctor probably has the results already by one month of age. If your baby is growing and thriving well, your baby is likely to be good because of his temperament and not due to any underlying medical condition. You do not have to worry.

256. *I'm concerned about our two-month-old's behavior. She cries all the time unless I pick her up, and only then does she stop. She wants to be glued to me day and night, and I can't get anything done. What am I doing wrong?*

You are not doing anything wrong. Remember, babies fuss because of their own temperament, not because of your mothering abilities. An understanding of what we call the *need-level* concept may help you understand why your baby wants to be held all the time. Every baby is born with a level of need in order to thrive to her maximum potential. Most babies also are born with a temperament which corresponds to their level of need. If yours needs a high level of holding in order to thrive, she fusses in order that her needs get met. Remember, babies are programmed for surviving and thriving, not to be convenient. Suppose your baby had a high level of need to be held but was not endowed with the corresponding temperament to demand to be held. She may not thrive to her full potential. Think of your baby not as a fussy baby but as a high-need baby. This is a kinder term and more positively describes her temperament.

Here are some survival tips. The key is to match the need level of the baby with the giving level of the parents. First, change your mind-set about how babies really are. We are often led to think of them as "down babies," i.e., lying quietly in a crib most of the time, gazing passively at dangling mobiles, and being picked up at regular intervals to be cared for, changed and fed, and then put down again. This is an unrealistic behavioral profile of even an average baby, and certainly of a high-need baby. "Up babies" need to be held most of the time and put down to sleep or allowed free-style floor movements at regular intervals. Get a sling-type baby carrier and learn to wear your baby (see questions 37, 38 for tips on the art of wearing your baby). This allows you to get things done but at the same time accommodates your baby's need to be held. Finally, you *are* getting something done. You are doing the most important job in the world—mothering a human being.

257. *Our three-month-old hates his car seat. Every time I try to put him in it he screams. As a result I seldom go anywhere and I'm beginning to feel housebound. Help!*

Above all, don't be tempted to travel without your baby safely secured in the car seat, even though he cries. Safety comes first. Here are some suggestions on having both safe and pleasant car travel: If possible, time your car travel when the baby needs to nap, since oftentimes babies fall asleep in the car seat after a few minutes of driving. Take a few minutes before you travel to relax your baby with a soothing massage and a cuddle-walk. Sit in the car for a few minutes and cuddle and talk to your baby before placing him in the car seat. Make sure he's not hungry or out-of-sorts. If he still hates the car seat, get him used to this "special seat" (a term you can use for the older infant) by sitting next to him in the backseat while someone else drives. When he starts to fuss, lean over and comfort him while you are both still secured in your seat belts. This works well in our family.

As a last resort, breastfeeding a baby in a car seat can be mastered. Tuck your legs up underneath yourself on the automobile seat and lean over and breastfeed your baby. (Warn your husband that you are going to try this so he is not surprised at the scene in the rearview mirror!) Feeding the baby in the car seat also works for bottle-feeding mothers.

258. *I am puzzled about our two-year-old's insistence on having things her own way. If she wants a peanut butter sandwich and I use the wrong type of bread, she has a fit. Is this behavior normal?*

Yes. For example, just the other day our two-year-old wanted some ice cream. Since it was a warm day and her request seemed reasonable, I gave her some ice cream, but neglected to also supply her favorite spoon. She got very upset until I recognized that she wanted her own spoon, the one she was accustomed to. Perhaps the reason why two-year-olds exhibit such meticulous attention to detail and a

limited tolerance for alternatives is best explained by looking at how a child's memory develops. Consider a child's
memory like the grooves in a record. During the first few
years children develop patterns of association: White bread
goes with brown peanut butter and red jelly; ice cream goes
in a certain dish with a certain spoon; mustard goes with
hot dogs and ketchup with hamburgers. Some children form
deep patterns of association, but do not yet have the mental
ability to realize that some alternatives are just as good or
even better. Perhaps in their developing minds the ice
cream may not taste as good from another spoon. Respect
this behavior as a developmental nuisance and do not get
into frustrating hassles or consider this a conflict of wills.
Don't feel that you are giving in and losing control if you
play this trivial association game. This is a passing stage
and your child will, within a year, be able to accept alternatives more easily.

You will also notice this behavior with dressing habits.
Your two-year-old may insist upon wearing a certain shirt
with a certain pair of pants even though they are obviously
mismatched. Experienced parents have learned to ride with
the flow of these humorous demands and try to anticipate
what their infants' associations are and match them. Take
a humorous approach to these bizarre behaviors of early
childhood—they soon will pass.

259. *Our one-year-old still sucks his thumb. We have a
history of orthodontic problems in our family, and I'm worried about this becoming a habit and affecting his teeth.
How can I stop it?*

Sucking is a natural instinct for infants. Even prenatal
babies suck their thumbs in the womb. Thumb sucking satis-
fies an infant's need for sucking. It soothes sore gums during
teething and helps the infant derive pleasure from his body
parts. As the sucking need diminishes toward the end of
the first year, some babies retain thumb or finger sucking
as a normal method of using their body parts to obtain

pleasure or relaxation. Infancy is a period of needing and finding security, and sucking is one of the symbols of this secure phase.

It is unlikely that at one year your child is harming his teeth by thumb sucking, since they are probably not developed enough to be made crooked by habitual thumb sucking. However, it can lead to an unbreakable habit later on and orthodontic problems may result.

At one year we would not advise you to discourage thumb sucking when your baby is doing it, but following are some suggestions on lessening his *need* to suck his thumb. Studies show that the lowest incidence of thumb sucking occurs in infants who are allowed to nurse off to sleep at their mothers' breasts. Going off to sleep is often when thumb sucking occurs, since sleep may induce a regressive behavior state, reminding the infant of earlier behaviors such as sucking. If babies have developed a mind-set that comfort equals nursing from another person, especially when going off to sleep, they are less likely to reach for their thumb. By the way, if you are breastfeeding you'll be glad to know, because of your family history of orthodontic problems, that long-term breastfeeding (past two years) can significantly lessen the severity of future dental misalignment and lower the amount of corrective work needed.

An older child may occasionally return to the comforts of thumb sucking to handle insecurity. Thumb sucking bothers adults more than infants. Parents should not always interpret it as a sign of parental failure and think, "Why should my child be insecure enough to need a crutch like his thumb?" Some children need to suck more than others and continue it well into childhood. We feel that, for many children, the ability to use their body parts for self-gratification is a sign of strength rather than weakness. Thumb sucking usually causes no orthodontic problems under three years of age. Beyond this age, however, persistent thumb sucking, especially at night, puts a large amount of negative pressure in the mouth and pulls on the front teeth and can result in protrusion of the upper teeth and pushing back of the lower teeth, causing an overbite.

If your child is old enough to be harming his teeth by thumb sucking, he should be old enough to understand that thumb sucking is harming his teeth. In our experience, mittens, restraints, or foul-tasting paints on the thumb do not work. Instead, talk to your child. Help him verbalize his feelings during what may be a stressful time. Try giving him an alternative to thumb sucking such as a large cuddle toy (a large teddy bear that he can get his arm around and thus cannot reach his thumb). If your pediatrician or dentist is concerned that habitual thumb sucking is causing orthodontic problems and the previously suggested methods aren't working, try the following: one, a behavior therapist who teaches your child alternative methods of comfort other than thumb sucking; and two, orthodontic appliances made by your dentist which protect the teeth during the thumb sucking and eventually discourage it.

260. *Our three-month-old cries a great deal of the time. My relatives are constantly advising me to let her cry it out, but I just can't. They tell me that crying is good for her lungs and that I am going to spoil her if I pick her up every time she cries. I just can't let her cry; it bothers me too much. Am I wrong?*

No, you are right—very right! You are doubly bothered, bothered by erroneous advice of your relatives and bothered by your baby's cry. Because your question is one of the most commonly asked yet most poorly answered, we are going to give you a very thorough and well-researched answer. A baby's cry is her language, designed for her survival and the development of the parent. Babies do not cry to annoy or to manipulate. They cry to signal a need. Parents, especially mothers, are naturally designed to respond to a baby's cry, not restrain themselves. For example, in experiments in which mothers were monitored by electronic sensing devices, when they heard their baby's cry (especially when they saw their babies crying) the following physiologic changes occured: The blood flow to the breasts increased, accompanied by a biological urge to pick up and comfort the baby. You're physiologically programmed to respond and not to restrain yourself. It is easy for someone else to advise you to let your baby cry. They are not physiologically wired to your baby—you are.

Your baby's cry is designed to bother you, thus guaranteeing a response and insuring that their needs of the young will be met. Alfred Lord Tennyson wrote:

But what am I?
An infant crying in the night,
An infant crying for the light
And with no language but a cry.

In the first few months of life a baby's needs are greatest and her skills to communicate these needs are least effective; she cannot tell us in plain language what she needs. To fill this gap in time in which she is unable to communicate clearly, she has been given a language we call a cry. There is probably no other sound that has been studied as extensively as the infant cry. Scientists have long been fascinated by the way the sound of a tiny infant can compel all within earshot to come to attention. Engineers who have extensively studied the infant cry describe it as a "perfect signal"—disturbing enough to alert the care giver to attend to the baby and stop the cry, but not so disturbing that it provokes an avoidance response.

The reason your baby's cry bothers you—and it should—is that you are a sensitive mother. Responding to her cry according to your intuition and not according to third-party advice allows you to develop your sensitivity. In counseling new parents on developing comforting skills, we have two goals: to mellow the temperament of the baby and improve the sensitivity of the parents. Promptly and appropriately responding to your baby's cry achieves both of these goals. I worry when a parents says, "My baby's cry doesn't bother me." I red-tag that baby's chart because I know a fundamental breakdown in baby–parent communication is beginning.

Concerning the wrongheaded advice—"It's good for her lungs"—studies show absolutely no beneficial effects of crying and certainly not of prolonged crying. In studies done on crying episodes without maternal response, babies' heart rates went up to worrisome levels, and the oxygen in the blood was diminished. As soon as these crying infants were soothed, their cardiovascular systems rapidly return to normal.

Concerning "spoiling," recent medical evidence goes against this theory. Babies whose cries earned prompt responses early in infancy actually cry less later on as they develop non-crying means of communicating their needs. They develop other body language. Both science and experience are finally turning the tide from the school of the restrained response to the nurturant response. Continue to follow your instinct—it won't fail you.

261. *Our two-year-old is still sleeping with us and still enjoys night nursing. We have all enjoyed this arrangement, but I feel it is now time to wean him from my breast and from our bed. Any suggestions?*

Weaning should occur when one or both members of the nursing and sleeping pair are ready, and it sounds as though you are. Since your toddler probably will not wean from your breast at night as long as he sleeps within close nursing distance to you, try the following: Have your husband sleep next to your child on a futon or mattress in his own room. Warn your husband that this will be one of the most difficult tasks he has ever done, but to persist. It may take several weeks. Dad will be forced to learn creative comforting measures that will enable the baby to get back to sleep. Be prepared for your baby to initially be furious at having to settle for his father's comfort rather than the breast to which he has long grown accustomed to expect. However, each night your baby will get more used to his father's comforting measures when he awakens and eventually will begin to sleep longer stretches, after which your husband will no longer have to sleep with him.

Remember, weaning implies substituting one form of nourishment (either emotional or nutritional) with another. Basically you are substituting dad at night for mom, or substituting one person for another. If your baby has been enjoying nighttime breastfeeding for two years, he probably will not settle for the much overrated nighttime teddy bear. He may still need a person to sleep with a bit longer.

If at some point in this weaning program you realize negative behaviors cropping up in your baby's daytime (e.g., anger or clinginess), you may need to back off and proceed more slowly. A good book to read concerning nursing an older baby is *Mothering Your Nursing Toddler*, available through La Leche League (see Appendix, page 280).

262. *Our two-year-old is still sleeping with us and doesn't seem to want to give up this arrangement. Quite frankly, neither do we. My mother-in-law says that we're going to be sorry that we let her into our bed because she'll never want to leave. Is she right?*

Yes and no. Yes, she may not want to leave your bed for a long time, but she will eventually want her own bed. Look at this arrangement from your child's point of view. If you enjoy any social relationship you don't want to give it up. If you enjoy your marriage you don't get a divorce. If you enjoy your job you don't quit. When a baby enjoys where she sleeps she is not going to want to settle for a less enjoyable sleeping arrangement. However, like all other weaning situations, children do eventually wean from the parents' bed, usually by the third or fourth year. We advise you to enjoy the present, since it is obviously working for you, and don't worry about the future. Children live in the present; perhaps adults occasionally should too.

263. *Our eleven-month-old son is starting to scream at the drop of a hat! It's embarrassing in restaurants, and I don't know how to handle this behavior. Is this the start of bad temper?*

No, he's just found his voice. This behavior, though common and normal in pre-verbal children, can be embarrassing in public places where you probably feel that people are wondering why you can't control your child. The reason for this vocal behavior is that once babies find their voice they like to exercise it. They take great delight in the pitch and volume of the new sounds they can produce and in the instant attention it gets from everyone within earshot. These are usually happy sounds, but can be quite disturbing.

Try to determine what triggers these vocal outbursts. They usually occur when a child is hyperstimulated or bored, or in a situation in which he wants attention. Here is how to modulate his screaming: When he screams, talk very softly back to him so that you model to him which language is pleasant and which sounds you enjoy. Make a mental note of what situations precede the outbursts of screaming, and try to distract him into other activities before screaming occurs. You *can* teach an eleven-month-old when screaming is and is not acceptable. When our one-year-old, Matthew, started screaming we taught him where he could acceptably scream. When he gave overtures that he was about to begin his screaming behavior, we took him outside along with the admonition, "Only screaming on the grass." We would let him stand in the yard and scream, sometimes doing it together just for fun! Gradually it sank in that he could scream outdoors. By the time he was sixteen months he was able to communicate with gestures and a few words, and the screaming behavior subsided.

264. *Our fifteen-month-old baby still enjoys breastfeeding. As soon as I sit down, she pounces on my lap and wants to nurse. Is this normal behavior, and what should I do?*

Yes, this *is* normal behavior, but too much of a good thing may be trying at times. Here's how you can get a few moments of peace away from your demanding toddler: First, it helps to understand why your toddler behaves this way. The atmosphere of nursing is one of the most pleasurable interactions of infancy, and it is the nature of toddlers (and adults, for that matter) to want to repeat those interactions which are most satisfying. When you sit in a place such as a rocking chair, which your baby has learned to associate with nursing, she clicks into a mental image of her nursing on your lap. The most repetitive and pleasant mental images are also those that are easiest to retrieve when given the slightest trigger. As much as possible, avoid sitting in those familiar places and in the usual position which reminds your baby of the nursing position or location. You also might try the technique called "scrambling" (a term used by a computer-engineer friend who has developed an ingenious variety of distraction techniques to relieve his wife of the incessant demands of their clinging toddler). As soon as your baby gives you nursing overtures—looks at you with the "I want to nurse" facial expression, moves toward you, and is about to pounce—you or your husband should quickly distract her into some other exciting activity. For example, pick up her favorite toy and exclaim, "Look what I have!" Some toddlers are more easily sidetracked than others into an alternative activity. Lessening the normal clinging behavior of toddlers can be accomplished by replacing previous mind-sets with new, exciting, equally pleasurable experiences.

265. *I'm a committed father, and since my wife also has a career outside the home, I help as much as possible with the care of our ten-month-old baby. However, diaper changing is such a wrestling match with our protesting young son that I dread this particular chore. Any advice?*

As a father of seven who has logged many hours of diaper-changing matches, I can offer some practical tips to change your wrestling match into a playful interaction. Most babies protest diaper changing because they feel restrained being placed on their backs and required to lie passively while some powerful person hovers over them, applying cold water and then tight pants on sensitive skin! Use a time-tested principle of playful interaction called a setting event. Reserve his favorite game for diaper changes. Just before you begin, sing his favorite song, use his favorite facial gestures and body-touch games, (e.g., walking your fingers over his tummy), and then begin changing his diaper. He will associate diaper changing with this playtime with you, as if he clicks into the playful interaction and only incidentally gets his diaper changed as part of the whole deal. We hung a black-and-white mobile over the changing area, so that the baby focused on the mobile while I worked on the other end. Use warm water and a soft washcloth to cleanse him. Also, babies prefer to lie on a blanket on the floor near the sink, and have you kneel during a diaper change rather than being placed on a hard surface such as a counter top next to the sink. Follow the diaper change with a special playful interaction that you reserve just for these times so that the baby learns to anticipate what event follows the changing. Babies often squirm less during this period of quiet anticipation.

266. *Our two-year-old is starting to whine and it drives me nuts. She has such a nice voice when she talks normally. Should I ignore her whining? How can I stop it?*

Tell your child just what you told us—she has such a nice voice most of the time, whining is irritating. Use language she can understand. It seldom helps to ignore whining, but this may work with some children. Frankly, I feel that pretending you don't hear is confusing to an intelligent child who knows that you do hear her. On the contrary, children should learn what kind of language gets the most pleasant response from their listeners. You want to convey to your toddler that whining is not one of the preferred means of communication. When she addresses you in her normal voice, come back with an *immediate and pleasant* response so that she learns that her regular voice is the one that gets the best response. As soon as she starts to whine, quickly get her to change communication channels by saying, "(toddler's name), you have such a nice voice. Use your regular voice." Eventually you can simply return the address by saying, "Regular voice" (always addressing her by name). Some impulsive beginning speakers need frequent reminders to help them click in to the voice which gets them the quickest response. Whining normally lessens as speech fluency increases, as if the toddler better enjoys her regular voice and the better response she gets. Remember, children whine because it *works*. Teach your child that his regular voice "works."

267. *Our seven-month-old is a very happy baby and seems very attached to me, in a secure sort of way. However, he is fearful when other people approach him. This is embarrassing to me and somewhat disappointing to his grandparents, for he often cries when they approach him. How can I help him warm up to others?*

This behavior is called *stranger anxiety* and is normal between six and nine months of age. Most babies experience a period of stranger anxiety during the first couple of years. Some sensitive babies show signs of it as early as four months, while others are not fearful of strangers until toddlerhood. Typically, your baby clings to you, looks fearful, or even cries when someone unfamiliar to him approaches.

Here's how to minimize your baby's stranger anxiety. Remember, he regards you as the standard by which he measures everyone else. If the approaching stranger is okay to you, he must be okay to the baby. Quickly greet the approaching stranger while he is still some distance away. Then, still keeping some distance from the stranger, continue the joyful dialogue with a welcoming smile. (Moving gradually from the familiar to the unfamiliar is an important strategy at this age.) Your baby begins to form a concept

about the stranger based on your reaction. Prepare signifi-
cant "strangers"—grandparents, good friends—not to be too
aggressive with your baby but to let you set the stage so
that eventually the baby will come to them. Suggest they
play with one of his favorite toys or an unfamiliar toy that
will engage his interest. This may help him warm up to a
stranger who, incidentally, possesses the toy that he wants.

268. *Our eight-month-old baby is very sensitive. She cries
every time I put her down and walk into the next room. I
can't seem to leave her without her getting upset. We have
had a very close relationship, but could I have made her
too dependent on me?*

Separation anxiety, which begins in most babies around
seven to eight months and may last until around fifteen to
eighteen months, is a common and perhaps healthy behavior. We developed our own theory about separation anxiety
as we watched our baby crawl across the room. Every five
feet or so she would turn her head and check to see if mom
and dad were there. At this age she would often cry if she
did not find us of if she saw us walking out of the room.
Separation anxiety seems to begin when a baby develops
the locomotive skills needed to move away from her parents.
Although your baby now has the power to initiate a separation, she is very fearful of it. It could be that separation
anxiety keeps a baby from drifting beyond her parent's
protective influence and thus, it has survival benefits. Respect
your baby's separation anxiety. Make continuous voice contact when you are out of sight of her. Most babies of seven
or eight months have not yet developed object or person
permanence; this means that if they cannot see or hear you,
they think that you no longer exist. Mental permanence usually
does not develop until a later stage, when a baby develops
sufficient memory to realize that you can continue to exist
out of her sight. Even if you are in another room, periodically
call out her name and reassure her, "Mommy's here."
    One day I watched our baby, Matthew, through a crack

in the bathroom door after I had walked away and left him. He had watched me leave and continued to gaze at the space where he had last seen me, wondering and expecting me to reappear. Without waiting for Matthew to cry anxiously, I reassured him with the sound of my voice. As soon as he heard me speak, he resumed his play, as if he realized he no longer had to worry about my disappearance.

Separation anxiety teaches us an important concept about weaning: The infant should separate from the mother and not the mother from the baby. Your baby will not separate from you completely until she has the cognitive ability to develop a mental image of you and, as it were, take you with her. Locomotive and mental capabilities develop together and are mutually dependent on each other. They work together beautifully to promote a gradual weaning. Researchers have used the term *hatching* to describe the process of a baby going from oneness to separateness.

269. *We are really enjoying our new baby. We carry him a lot, take him with us most of the time, and pick him up every time he cries. But our friends tell us that we are going to spoil him, or that we are creating a dependency and he will never want to be away from us. I feel right about our parenting, but I guess I need some reassurance that we are doing the right thing. Can you give it to me?*

You are doing right! It is very important that parents feel right about their parenting style. If it is working and you feel right about it, then the particular parenting style that you have chosen is right for your family. We would like to put the spoiling theory on the shelf—to spoil forever. Spoiling means leaving something alone, such as putting fruit on the shelf to spoil. You do not spoil a baby by developing a close relationship with your baby. The attachment style of parenting does not mean overindulgence or inappropriate dependency. The possessive parent or the hovering mother is one who keeps an infant from doing what he needs to do because of her own needs. This style has a detrimental affect on the development of both the infant and the parent. Attachment differs from dependency. Attachment enhances development; dependency may hinder it.

You will be happy to know that current research has finally "spoiled" the spoiling theory. Perhaps an explanation of what we call our deep-groove theory will give you a clearer understanding of the meaning of a healthy dependency and attachment. Suppose the strength of parent–infant attachment is represented by the depth of the groove that is recorded in a baby's mental record. Early theories of infant behavior that popularized the idea of spoiling claimed that an infant that was strongly attached to his mother would never get out of this deep groove to become independent and explore his world. Experiments have shown the opposite to be true. The most securely attached infants, the ones with the deepest grooves, actually showed less anxiety when separated from their mothers to explore toys in the same room. They periodically checked in with their mothers (returning to the groove) for reassurance that it was okay to explore. The mother seems to add energy to the infant's exploration. Since the infant does not need to waste effort worrying about whether his mother is there, he can use that energy for exploration. An infant with a more shallow attachment groove may not be able to avail himself of this energy-conservation system. Studies have shown that infants who develop a secure attachment to their mothers during the first year are better able to tolerate separation from them when they are older. Infants raised by the attachment style of parenting you are practicing actually turn out to be sensitive children who are much easier to discipline. As one sensitive mother of a well-disciplined child proudly exclaimed, "He's not spoiled, he's perfectly fresh!"

270. *Our two-year-old is a head banger. She doesn't seem angry and seems to enjoy it. Can she hurt herself?*

Usually not. Head banging is a surprisingly common behavior. Equally surprising is the fact that children seldom hurt themselves by banging their heads. Like most undesirable behavior, head banging bothers the parents more than the children. In trying to discourage any undesirable behavior in children, try to determine what triggers this behavior. Make a list of the circumstances which provoke head banging. Is she tired? bored? in a confining place such as a crib? When you have determined what situations provoke this behavior, try to change them as much as possible. If you sense that your child simply likes feeling the impact on her head, play the "bump the heads" game. Hold your child standing on a table in front of you so that your heads are the same height and *gently* and playfully bump foreheads. This behavior will soon disappear as your child finds more exciting things to do.

271. *Our twenty-month-old has frequent temper tantrums. At the end of these bouts he's a wreck and I am too. Sometimes I feel helpless. How should I handle these tantrums?*

You cannot "handle" your child's tantrums. You can only understand and support them. Temper tantrums are not abnormal. They do not mean that your child is basically disturbed or has received ineffective parenting. These tantrums should not always be considered misbehavior. Two inner feelings prompt most temper tantrums: Your child has an intense curiosity and desire to accomplish an activity, but often his desire is greater than his capability. This leads to intense frustration, which is released in a healthy, outward tantrum. Second, newly found power and desire for "bigness" propel him toward a certain action, when suddenly someone from above, especially someone he loves, descends upon him with a no. Acceptance of an outside force contrary to his strong will may be very difficult. He cannot handle this conflict without a fight. He wants to be big, but reality tells him how small he is. He is angry but does not yet have the language to express his anger, so he expresses it through actions. Your child does not yet have the ability to handle emotions with reason, so he chooses to cope with his emotions by an outward display which we call tantrums.

Try to achieve a balance in helping your child. Too much interference deprives him of the ability to release his inner tensions, whereas not enough support leaves him to cope all by himself without the reserves to do so effectively. The advice to ignore it is poor. Ignoring any behavior problem in your child deprives him of a valuable support resource and deprives you of an opportunity to improve your rapport with your child. Simply being available during a tantrum gives your child the needed crutch. Temper tantrums bring out the best in intuitive mothering and fathering. If your child is losing control and needs help to regain it, often a few soothing words or a little help (I'll untie the knot and then you can put on the shoe) may put him back on the road to recovery. If he has chosen an impossible task, distract him or channel him into more easily achievable play. Keep your arms extended and your attitude accepting.

If your child is strong-willed, he may lose complete control of himself during a tantrum. It often helps to simply hold him firmly but lovingly and explain, "You are angry and you have lost control. I am holding you because I love you." You may find that after a minute or two of struggling to free himself, he relaxes in your arms, as if to thank you for rescuing him. Fortunately, toddlers have a magnificent resilience for recovering from temper tantrums. They usually do not sulk for long, and a properly supported temper tantrum usually wears off quickly in the child (but may leave parents exhausted). Temper tantrums are self-limiting. Your child does not like these feelings, and as soon as he has developed the language to express his emotions you will find that this disturbing behavior subsides.

272. *Our eighteen-month-old holds her breath during a temper tantrum until she almost passes out. This is very scary for her and for me. How can I stop this behavior?*

Breath-holding spells are the most frightening form of temper tantrum. During the rage of a tantrum a child may hold her breath, turn blue, become limp, and even faint. In some children the breath-holding episode resembles a convulsion and becomes even more alarming to the already worried parent. Fortunately, most children who hold their breath do resume normal breathing just as they are on the brink of passing out. Even those children who faint quickly resume normal breathing before harming themselves. Make a list of what situations trigger this breath-holding behavior. Usually it occurs during a period of intense frustration in the impulsive child whose desires are greater than her capabilities. Try to intervene and help your child *before* she loses control. Either help her complete the task that is frustrating her, or redirect her energies into a more easily achievable activity. Breath-holding episodes usually stop when a child is between two and two and a half, and is old enough to express her frustrations verbally.

273. *Our two-year-old throws a tantrum in the most embarrassing places, usually when I take him shopping. It's so bad I'm staying home more and more. I'm beginning to feel housebound. Help?*

When your child disintegrates in public places, your embarrassment makes it often difficult to consider his feelings first. Your first thought is more likely to be, "What will people think of me as a mother?" Tantrums often occur when we impose unrealistic expectations on a child. To expect a curious toddler to be a model of obedience in a supermarket, where he is surrounded by a smorgasbord of tempting delights, may be asking too much. Try these tips to enjoy going out with your child: First, plan your outings at the time of the day when your child's behavior is the best, usually in the mornings. Late mornings and late afternoons are usually the time when a toddler's behavior begins to deteriorate, primarily because he is tired and hungry. Children who are overly tired and hungry are especially prone to mood changes and temper tantrums. Be sure your child is well rested and well fed before you go out. It helps to take along a bag full of his favorite nutritious nibbles and toys.

Tantrums often occur in public places when your child senses that you are not tuned into him. He resorts to a tantrum in order to break through to you. Try a "fun trip" to the supermarket. Put your child into the shopping cart and go up and down the aisle pointing out things to him and letting him help put nonbreakable items from the shelf into the cart. The purpose of this trip is primarily to have fun and not to shop. Do this several times and you will be setting your child up to regard shopping with his mother as a fun activity and not a restraining and boring time. If he still hates to go to certain places where you have to go, combine your shopping trip with a fun activity such as stopping by the park for a few minutes of play before or after your trip. This sets your child up to associate your shopping trip with some pleasant activity for him.

274. *Our two-year-old likes to bang things, especially utensils on her plate during dinner. This is especially embarrassing when we have guests over. How can I handle this behavior?*

Between one and two years of age, banging with sticks is a normal developmental achievement. The child is learning she can extend her reach with the use of sticks, and she is learning contingency play—the sound produced is contingent upon how she bangs the utensils. Here's how we have mellowed this dinnertime noise in our toddler: Place a small, pleasant-sounding drum and wooden drumstick next to your child's plate. Let her play the drum for a few minutes before the meal begins. This will temporarily satisfy her desire to bang. If she starts to pick up and bang the utensils, quickly redirect her activity by saying, "Only hit the drum." Also, plastic utensils may help.

In redirecting undesirable behavior in children, we use the principal of shaping rather than controlling a child's behavior. We have found, as have other experienced parents, that understanding why your child does certain things helps you develop your intuitive powers of learning how to read your child. In the example of banging at the dinner table, you could simply grab the utensils from your child and shout, "Don't bang." You succeed in stopping this one incident, but that's all you've gained. By redirecting a child's energy into more creative behavior, you develop your own creative parenting, and your child gains a bit of emotional maturity. Don't feel that you are a weak parent or compromising. In fact, you are more in charge of your child, taking the extra time and effort to shape her behavior rather than simply stopping it. Shaping implies using discipline techniques to work through your child's personality. Controlling implies that you are first considering your own personality, and making your child conform to this. Controlling leads to frustration and lessens your enjoyment of your child; shaping puts you more in harmony with her and leads to the ultimate goal of this book—to help you better understand and enjoy your child.

275. *Our two-year-old hates to share. He grabs and holds onto his toys when a friend comes over to play. How can I teach him to share?*

Toy squabbles are to be expected, since possession means ownership at this age. Have other children bring over a few toys of their own when they come to visit. Capitalize on a natural desire of children to play with another child's toys. As your child grabs a toy, another child will grab his toy. He will learn to give a toy to get a toy. If the children are still having trouble sharing, try the time method. Set an alarm or stove buzzer for five minutes and announce that one child gets one toy and another child gets the other for five minutes. When the buzzer goes off, they exchange toys. You will probably find that when the timer goes off, the children don't want each other's toys anymore and they're off to another activity.

Parents can model sharing for their child. When he

wants something you have—and they usually do—comply. "Yes, Daddy likes to share; I feel good when I share my things with you." This attitude will impress on your child the value of sharing; in addition, since the interchange was initiated by the child, it will sink in better than a whole speech on sharing. Capitalize on the normally egocentric child's desire to feel good. The concept of "when you do good (share) you feel good" may help sharing become a habit.

276. *Our two-year-old is becoming extremely negative. She seems to always want to do the opposite thing from what I want her to do. When I ask her to come to me, she runs the other way. How should I handle this?*

Wisely! Parents sometimes have difficulty telling the difference between defiance and a growing child normally exerting his will. Your child is probably not feeling, "I won't," but instead, "I don't want to." It is your job as a parent to help her "want to." Developing a strong will is part of the normal growth of a toddler. That is what helps her get up from a fall and keep going, explore new avenues, and develop into an independent person. However, your child also needs to know that you are in charge. Defiance, meaning persistently ignoring a reasonable request, should not go unrecognized and undisciplined. The late Dr. Selma Fraiberg, author of the classic child psychology book *The Magic Years*, wrote this about defiant toddlers, "The toddler exerts a normal declaration of independence but does not have a desire to overthrow the government."

277. *Our two-year-old seems hyperactive, I can't tell whether this is abnormal or if he's just a very active little boy. When should I worry?*

Here are some guidelines to help you determine whether your child's hyperactivity is normal and needs to be accepted or abnormal and needs to be shaped: Normally a very active child is happy, fun (although exhausting) to be around, does

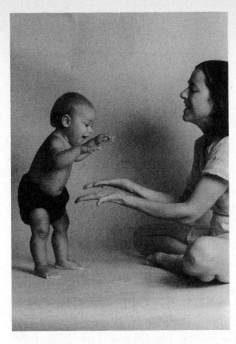

Playing "give me five" will defuse a baby's hitting.

not trigger many angry feelings in his parents, has a reasonable attention span (five to ten minutes) in one play activity, and is able to play reasonably well with other children without a great deal of anger or aggressive behavior. On the other hand, signs that your child's hyperactivity may be abnormal and in need of professional counseling are the following: He seems to operate from a constant feeling of anger; he is seldom fun to be with and you have frequent feelings of "I don't really like him," or "I look forward to being away from him"; with each passing month his behavior is becoming more disorganized and out of control; and your relationship with him and his relationship within the whole family is deteriorating.

In the former case, time, maturity, and a bit of organizing of your child's behavior may be all that is necessary. In the latter, he is not likely to grow out of *it* but to grow into more undesirable behavior. If this is the case, behavior modification is necessary and we suggest that you obtain professional counseling. (See question 278 for treatment of hyperactivity.)

278. *Our three-year-old has been diagnosed as a hyperactive child, and our doctor wants to put her on Ritalin. I don't like giving drugs to a child. Could you explain how this medication works? Is it safe?*

In carefully screened children, these medications to control hyperactivity are safe and effective. They are stimulants which in a hyperactive child work on the part of the brain that causes the child to be easily distracted. Their main purpose is to encourage more purposeful behavior. Parents are reluctant and physicians are cautious in using medications for behavioral modification. It often helps to consider the consequences of not using them. Is it fair to your child to withhold the benefit of a proven medication which may enable him to learn better and thus be a happier person? In our practice, we always caution parents not to rely completely on medication. Behavioral-modification medicine is only an adjunct to other forms of treatment, namely behavioral modification. However, in truly hyperactive children (also called attention deficit disorder, or ADD), behavioral modification alone is much less effective without the attention stimulating effects of medication.

Fortunately, children who show improved behavior on these medications do so within a few days to weeks. This is important since time is important to a developing child who cannot afford several years of unproductive behavior. Think of medication as an adjunct to behavioral modification, like setting your child's "behavioro-stat" to a point where she is more receptive to behavioral modification and learning.

In addition to medicines for hyperactivity, improved behavior results in some children after diet modification. Some children are highly vulnerable to the effects of junk food—namely highly sugared and artificially colored foods. A trial period off these junk foods may significantly improve your child's behavior. Food allergies can adversely affect a child's behavior, and an elimination diet may be necessary. Frequent grazing often lessens mood swings in a three-year-old hyperactive child, especially frequent grazing on nutritious food (for example, fruit may prevent blood sugar swings and steady her behavior). A strong dose of family harmony may also help improve your child's behavior. Family stress, marital stress, frequent absentee parents, frequent moves, sibling strife, and any other family situation which threatens a child's self-esteem may adversely affect her behavior.

279. *Our two-year-old is becoming stubborn, strong-willed, and defiant. She wants her own way all the time. Is this the terrible twos I hear about?*

The term *terrible twos* is one of the most unfair labels ever applied to babies. We prefer "terrific twos." An understanding of a normal two-year-old's growth and development will help you survive this passing stage. We believe that becoming strongwilled is a normal developmental trait which enables a toddler to become a child. It helps her get up after a fall, overcome obstacles in her quest to walk and run, and keep practicing and refining a developmental skill until she has mastered it. Also, around two years of age a child begins to develop a concept of self, hence, the "I do it myself" stage. This is a normal and necessary stage in order that the child separate and become gradually independent of her parents.

The term defiance may be overstated in most two-year-olds. Your daughter is probably not giving you the message "I won't," but rather "I don't want to." This message ties in with her emergence of the concept of self. It helps to give your strong-willed two-year-old choices. For example, our two-and-a-half-year-old son, Matthew, used to grab chocolate while waiting in the check-out line in the supermarket. Angrily grabbing the chocolate bar from him and putting it back on the rack only resulted in a temper tantrum and an exhausted mother and child. We have found it much easier to say, "Do you want Mommy to put it back or Matthew to put it back?" Giving choices to your child sends the message that you are in charge (the candy bar must go back), but that you also respect her will as to how to put it back. Using creative discipline with a two-year-old means developing a balance between an appreciation of the normal behavioral traits at this age and the need for your child to know that you are in charge.

280. *Our twenty-two-month-old seems so aggressive. He enjoys pushing other children around and I'm afraid he'll hurt someone. How can I lessen his aggression?*

First, be sure you understand the difference between being aggressive and being assertive. Aggressiveness means infringing on someone else's territory. Being assertive means protecting one's own turf. It does sound as if your child is truly being aggressive. Next, examine the models in your child's environment. Is he around a lot of aggressive children, learning that pushing and shoving is a way of life? A two-year-old begins to form his own "laws of the jungle" during social play. It is important that he be taught gentleness during play. Invite another child who you know is gentle but also fun and supervise the play interaction. If your child becomes aggressive, intervene by showing him how to hug and touch gently, not angrily or aggressively. Finally, take inventory of your child's overall emotional state. Is he angry? If so, try to determine why. Angry children have difficulty controlling their impulses, and this is often reflected in aggressive and impulsive behavior.

281. *Our two-and-a-half-year-old throws a tantrum when it is time to leave the baby-sitter's. She gets so involved in what she is doing that I literally have to drag her away. Help!*

Children often become so intently involved in a play activity that they don't want to give it up without a fight. Here's how to lessen these departure hassles: If your child is intensely involved in one of her favorite activities, begin to wind up this activity at least five-to-ten minutes before departure time. To suddenly pick her up off her favorite riding toy guarantees a protest. Gradually close out the activity by appropriate departure gestures, such as: "Bye-bye truck, bye-bye boy (name of friend), bye-bye blocks," etc. By encouraging your child to use these departure gestures you are helping the normally strong-willed child to close out her own activities.

282. *Our eighteen-month-old has begun biting. I'm embarrassed to take him to a play group because of this offensive habit and I'm loosing friends whose toddlers have been bitten. How can I stop this behavior?*

There are as many theories about biting as there are teeth. Biting usually occurs between the ages of eighteen months and two and a half years in a pre-verbal child, and lessens when he can effectively communicate his feelings with language rather than with aggressive actions. Because your child's mouth and hands are his first tools of communication, biting and hitting are forms of communication to him. However, he soon learns that this is undesirable behavior by others' negative reactions. We suggest the following tips to stop biting: Try to determine why your child bites, and the circumstances in which he bites. When approaching any undesirable behavior, first consider the feeling and the cause behind the action rather than the action itself. Is your child tired, hungry, angry, or just plain bored? Make a diary of the circumstances surrounding the biting, and avoid these circumstances as much as possible. Biting often occurs when a child is tired or in close quarters with another child and a play conflict arises. If through experience you can detect the usual circumstances which prompt your child to bite, attempt to act before these circumstances arise. Biters should always be supervised. If a child consistently hurts another child by biting and scratching, it is often wise to separate these children. This isolation teaches the biter a valuable social lesson. Biters seem to be the instant center of attention, and so biting may fulfill the craving for attention that's reinforcing this undesirable behavior. It is difficult to ignore biting, since someone is being hurt. However, if you think the biting represents a simple craving for attention, then the "ignore him" advice may be applicable. In general, ignoring undesirable behavior is an unwise approach.

In addition to hurting other children, biting is very hard on mothers. The mother of a biter is both disturbed and embarrassed; the mother of the bitee is naturally upset that her child has been hurt, and negative feelings between mothers often result. A good way to handle this problem is to discuss beforehand that your child is going through a biting stage, that you are concerned, and that he needs supervision. When he bites, remove him from the play group with the appropriate admonitions, such as, "Biting hurts, and it is wrong to hurt." Above all, do not bite your child back. You are a mature person and biting is an immature, undesirable act.

If you feel that your child really does not understand that biting hurts, and all of the above measures have failed, a technique that we and other parents have used successfully is to take your child's forearm and press it against his upper teeth, as if he is biting himself. This demonstrates that biting hurts. Do this immediately after he has bitten another child to show him that biting hurts.

When your child learns to talk better and can express his actions more in words than in deeds, you will notice that his biting behavior subsides. Persistent biting in a child over three with good verbal skills is a cause for concern, and you should seek professional counseling.

283. *Our daughter is entering those terrible twos and I wonder if I should spank her. Some of my relatives tell me that spanking is the way to discipline her, but my heart*

just isn't in it. I'm confused about the issue of spanking.
Can you clarify?

To spank or not to spank is currently the subject of much
debate among child-care writers. It has produced a flurry of
controversial books, magazine articles, TV programs, and
even legislation. Our own opinion about spanking is based
upon our experience as parents and health care professionals. The first point we would like to make is that it is
absolutely wrong to be mean and abusive toward a child or
to strike a child out of frustration, hostility, or anger. Second, spanking should never be a first resort in discipline. A
parent ought to strive to create the sort of attitude within
their child and atmosphere within their home that renders
spanking unnecessary. Third, spanking should be reserved
for major confrontations when a parent's authority is on the
line, for situations in which your child knowingly and will-
fully defies reasonable authority, and in which her safety is
an issue. For instance, spanking *may* be the only way to
teach a small child the danger of going into the street. The
child under three and a half years of age, however, is too
young to understand the process of spanking, and a child
that young needs to be under constant adult supervision
when there is a dangerous situation. Another situation that
may justify spanking would be the use and respect of fenced
swimming pools. These situations and others will come up
from time to time, but they are not part of everyday parent–
child interactions. Many parents who are using spanking to
discipline are doing it on a weekly, daily, or even hourly
basis. We see this as inappropriate and very damaging, a
situation where counseling is needed.

The longer we are in pediatric practice and the more
years we have spent as parents, the less enthused we are
about spanking. More often than not, spanking puts a distance between parent and child. In our family we have found
other disciplinary methods, such as time out and logical
consequences, to be much more effective.

It is unwise to give an absolute spank or never spank

dictum to parents. If spanking is even to be considered, there are important guidelines which *must* be understood (such as where to spank, with what, and how much, etc.) Such a crucial decision should not be made without study.

Every parent should also consider if there are specific risk factors in her family that affect her attitude towards spanking. Parents who are most likely not to abuse spanking show the following features: They have practiced the principles of attachment parenting all along, so that they know their children and their children feel trust rather than fear. They have children whose temperaments are generally easy going, who would need spanking very infrequently, if at all. The parents themselves were not spank-controlled as children.

Parents who are at high risk for spanking inappropriately and for abusing their child show the following features: They generally have shaky parent–child relationships, were themselves abused as children, have high-need children, find that spanking does not work, and are prone to impulsive anger. If you have any of these risk factors that might result in inappropriate spanking, we suggest you examine your entire parent–child relationship.

In our family, we have concluded the following concerning spanking:

1. We do not let any wrong behavior go undisciplined.
2. We are committed to create an attitude within our children and an atmosphere within our home that renders spanking unnecessary. Spanking, which actually is punishment, in general is a poor option in all the methods of discipline.
3. If in certain circumstances spanking seems to be the wisest direction, we are open to it.

In short, we really don't *want* to spank our children, so we are going to devote a lot of time and energy to remove the need for spanking.

One more point we'd like to make is that the two's are terrific, not terrible. Reading up on the development of the two-year-old and having appropriate expectations will be an important part of how you plan the discipline of this special little person.

284. *Our two-and-a-half-year-old is very hard to discipline. The harder I spank, the worse he gets. I am at my wit's end. I can't seem to get through to him. Help!*

Discipline is the most important aspect of parenting and perhaps the least well understood. There are no short and easy answers; we could write a book just to respond to this question. You are assuming that discipline equals spanking. Actually, discipline has nothing to do with spanking. The concept of discipline includes two basic ideas: instruction (teaching) and correction (chastening). Instruction takes place when all is well—your child is behaving. Correction takes place when there is a problem—your child is misbehaving. Instruction and correction are positive, forward-thinking, healthy, wholesome activities resulting in security for the child. Spanking, on the other hand, is punishment. It, like correction, takes place when there is misbehavior, but the similarity ends there. Spanking is negative, focusing on the past behavior committed. It carries an attitude of hostility, frustration, even possibly sadism, and tends to result in fear, unhealthy guilt, resentment, and possibly even rejection in the child. There is a very fine line between spanking as correction and spanking as abuse. We see spanking ultimately creating a distance between parent and child that may be difficult to bridge. Punitive actions have a vengeful quality, a feeling of "You're going to pay for this." Often the parent is thinking "He has to learn" or "I'll teach him." Teaching does not occur through punishment. The purpose of punishment is to inflict a penalty for misbehavior. If the child learns anything, it is not to get caught next time or that it is somehow right for big people to hurt little people (who must therefore be bad). The end result is that, as you say, the harder or more often you spank, the less it works. Or if it does, you have achieved a spank-controlled child rather than one who is learning the difference between right and wrong.

Your statement "the harder I spank, the worse he gets" gives you a clue that a change in disciplining technique is needed. Your child is probably operating more from a feeling of anger than of trust, especially if he has been spanked for a long time. Try a rebuilding program to regain his trust. Give him lots of hugs and kisses, touch, focused attention, eye-to-eye contact. Speak to him in a firm, "I'm in charge" voice but in a loving, respectful way. A two-and-a-half-year-old is a little person with big needs. He needs to know that you're in charge, but he also needs to trust you. A child who operates on the basis of mistrust is very hard to discipline.

The principals of attachment parenting form the best program for building or rebuilding trust. Discipline begins at birth—everything you do with your baby from day one fits either the category of teaching or of correcting, sometimes both (as, for example, when you are getting your new baby to breastfeed correctly—your first discipline situation). Over the months your baby learns trust because of your responsive parenting and when he turns two you are well on your way to having a child who is easy to discipline. Why? Because you know him so well (attachment develops this beautifully) and he trusts you so completely. He knows you are always there for him.

We strongly suggest that you learn more about the subject of discipline by reading some of the excellent books written on the subject. These are available through La Leche League International. You can write to them for a complete list of their recommended books. (See Appendix page 280, for LLLI address.)

We have often talked to parents in your situation, who have been spanking more and more and seeing it cause this same problem of distancing. At our suggestion they have decided to stop spanking their child, and they have reported back to us, excitedly, that things are so much better now that spanking is no longer a part of their lives.

285. *My thirteen-month-old used to be easy to look after, but now she's getting into everything. I watch my friends deal with their toddlers, and I see a lot of slapping of children's hands, angry voices, and tears. Is this what our relationship will be like soon?*

We can't think of one good reason why you would slap the hand of a child. Some of the usual causes given are electric outlets, the getting into all the cupboards, touching the antique vase, or even pulling baby sister's hair. There is a much more creative way to deal with these problems than hand slapping. Electric outlets can be covered, cupboards can be latched with safety hooks, antique vases can be removed to higher ground, and little ones can be taught how to treat their baby sisters gently.

A wise teacher of small children once told us that slapping a child's hand inhibits her drive to explore because the hand is her tool for exploration. In fact, most everything a child does with her hands is her exploring and learning about her world. Sometimes this behavior needs to be redirected into more constructive learning, but never should it be squelched by inflicting corporal punishment.

We often hear parents explaining how they smack their babies or toddlers on the mouth or face for screaming or otherwise misusing their voices. Remember, a slap to the face is the highest form of insult to any human being, no matter what her age. If corporal punishment is even considered, the only place on the child's body that should be spanked is the buttocks. And parents must remember that they can do just as much damage with what they say to their children and how they say it as they can do by physically abusing them. Verbal abuse, whether it be with the tone of voice or the actual words is a serious attack on your child's self-esteem.

How you deal with your toddler's energetic need to explore will determine whether you will have a terrible two or a terrific two. If you are constantly using the word no with your thirteen-month-old, you may find that this is the only word she has for you when she is two. Instead of always saying no, try saying "stop," or "not safe," or "come see Mama" and redirect her physical activity into something safer or more constructive.

You are right to be considering now what your relationship is headed for. Those early months of mobility and increasing independence require a lot of intensive one-on-one, moment-by-moment teaching. Your baby, after all, needs to know what is expected of her. Putting in the time now will give major payoffs when she's two. This is one of those times when you could very easily "spoil" your child by leaving her alone too much to learn for herself.

286. *Our twenty-month-old simply will not sit still to eat his meals. As soon as I put him in his high chair, he squirms to get out and meal times are an ordeal. Any suggestions?*

A creative feeding technique that we have used at this age is to put your baby on your lap, put his food (or your food) on your plate, and let him eat from it. Some toddlers eat better in the comfort of a parent's lap and from the parent's plate; others like the independence of their own high chair, dish, and utensils. This is a passing stage and soon he will want his own chair and plate. (See question 176 for more about feeding toddlers.)

8

SPECIAL
CONCERNS

T here are a variety of family circumstances which have a serious impact on the functioning of the family unit. The purpose of this chapter is to help parents and children fit together in less than ideal circumstances. During the writing of this book we gave birth to our seventh child, Stephen, a boy with special needs requiring a special kind of parenting. Stephen has Down's syndrome. During our parenting of Stephen we are realizing a very important principle of parenting—the *need-level* concept. Every child has a certain level of need, every parent a certain level of giving. A child with high needs requires constant giving, sometimes to the point that parents feel they can't give any more. At the same time, parents of high-need children naturally develop a higher level of parenting skills. With special children, this principle of mutual giving reaches its peak. As Stephen develops special skills, we develop special skills. Stephen is really bringing out the best in us. As one mother of a child with Down's syndrome in my practice wrote to us, "Stephen will add flashes of color to your lives that you never knew life could lack— wait and see." How true this has turned out to be.

287. *Our two-and-a-half-year-old enjoys imagining she is a dinosaur. Should I discourage these fantasies or go along with her?*

Go along. Enter into your child's fantasy world and enjoy it as she does. We have frequently used our children's fantasies to get them to behave the way that we would like. For example, "Dinosaurs eat their carrots," or "Dinosaurs like to take naps." It lets the child play her own game, and she is likely to do anything you ask.

While some fantasizing is normal for the young imaginative mind, too much may reflect hidden anxieties. A bored child may create a more interesting fantasy world. A child who is unhappy with or does not fit into the family situation may imagine a more compatible one. For example, following a move, a child may continue to imagine her previous friends. To cope with the loss of her pet, she may animate her rubber dog. Channel these fantasies into equally pleasant real-life situations, and the pretend creatures will soon pass away.

288. *I am afraid that someone may kidnap or molest our three-year-old. How can I protect her?*

Since you can't be with your child at every moment, teach her at an early age what to do to keep safe. Teach her about secrets. Tell her that she should tell you if anyone asks her to keep a secret. Teach her the difference between good secrets and bad secrets. If anyone gives her bad touches and asks her not to tell mommy and daddy, these are bad secrets. She should tell you about those. Good secrets are things like what someone is getting for a birthday present. Those are secrets she can keep. If anyone offers her money or candy or wants to take her picture, she should tell you, especially if that person tells her not to tell her parents. Build a trusting relationship with your child so that she feels comfortable telling you anything. We made the following bargain with our children beginning at age three: "Whatever you tell Mommy or Daddy, we will not get angry." Child molesters often tell their victims not to tell their parents and threaten them with the loss of parental love if they do. Your child should know that this will not happen.

Teach your child the meaning of "private parts" and that no one has the right to touch her in her private parts. Tell her that there are good touches and bad touches. Good touches make you feel safe. Bad touches make you feel frightened. Tell her that if anyone touches her in a way that makes her feel frightened, she should tell mommy or daddy. Teach your child what a stranger is: someone she does not know well. Uncle Harry and Aunt Nancy are not strangers, but anyone your child does not know well, even if it is someone from church or a classmate's parents, is a stranger. (Of course, she should know that if Uncle Harry touches her in a bad way she must tell you—abuse does not only come from strangers.)

Tell her never to get into a car with a stranger or show a stranger how to get somewhere if he stops and asks for directions, even if he says that he will take her to mommy or daddy. If someone other than a parent is picking up a child after school, the teacher should know about it. The child should walk home from school with other children. If she is lost in a store, she should not seek help from a stranger, but should go to a cash register and find a salesperson. Teach your child to run into a busy place where there are lots of people or into a neighbor's house or store if she is being followed. Tell her not to hide in a secluded place such as an alley or the woods. She should yell for help if a stranger is following her or grabbing her. Certainly, a three-year-old should not be left home alone, and older children should not let anyone into the house, for any reason. Be sure your child knows how to dial 911 or the operator for help in an emergency. Be aware of signs of sexual abuse in your children or in other children. These include sudden changes in behavior, fear of leaving you, fear of being washed during a bath, or a sudden fear of going to visit a previously trusted friend or relative. In most cases of sexual abuse, the abuser is someone the child already knows.

289. *We have a new baby and are worried about sudden infant death. Is there anything we can do to prevent it? How can we tell if our baby is at risk?*

Sudden infant death syndrome (SIDS), or crib death, is a worry for many families, but fortunately SIDS is still relatively uncommon and new research has helped identify some risk factors. The average incidence of SIDS is approximately one in four hundred babies. It is more prevalent in the winter months and usually occurs in infants between one and six months of age. The peak risk period is between two and four months. SIDS is rare after the age of eight months. In most cases of SIDS, the cause is unknown and researchers feel that there is more than one cause of death. The current theory is that most cases of SIDS are due to an abnormality in the part of the brain which automatically controls breathing. The following are situations which increase the risk of SIDS:

1. Premature babies.
2. Babies who have stop-breathing episodes during the first month, thought to have a temporary immaturity of their breathing regulating mechanisms.
3. Smoking and drug abuse by the mother.
4. A previous sibling who died of SIDS.

   This tragedy is seldom preventable because the cause is unknown. Current SIDS preventive research is aimed at identifying which infants are at risk. If your child is at risk, you should follow these steps: Consult with your doctor. Your baby may have a test called a twelve-to-twenty-four-hour sleep pneumogram. This specialized test is performed either in the newborn nursery or at home. Painless, this test consists of pasting wires on the baby's skin and recording changes in heart rate and breathing patterns during various stages of sleep.

If your baby shows any troublesome breathing or heart rate patterns on the sleep pneumogram, your doctor may suggest a home infant monitor—a lunch-box-size device which monitors the baby's heart rate and breathing during sleep, and sounds an alarm if abnormalities occur. As part of a home-monitoring program, parents are instructed in CPR and simple methods to restart normal breathing (which sometimes merely requires gently awakening the baby). Monitoring is usually discontinued after the risk period is over—between eight and twelve months of age. Further information regarding SIDS can be obtained from the National Sudden Infant Death Foundation, 300 South Michigan Avenue, Chicago, IL 60604, (312) 663-0650.

290. *Our new baby was born with Down's syndrome. We are devastated and are having a hard time coping. Help!*

The birth of a handicapped child is initially devastating for parents. The baby you expected is not the baby you got. Here are some tips on how you and your special baby can bring out the best in each other:

1. Join one of the many support groups composed of parents of Down's syndrome children. The best support is always from parents who have gone through similar situations as yours, have coped and thrived, and are able to share their experiences with you.
2. Don't compare. You have a special baby who will not develop like most other babies. If you try to compare yours with others you will be continually frustrated and disappointed. Your baby will have his own unique developmental milestones. You will experience joy at each one, although they may not be as clear-cut and on the same timetable as those of other babies.
3. Focus on the special qualities of your baby rather than on what he is missing when compared with other babies. One of the rewarding features of Down's syndrome babies is that they seem to generally be very happy babies, as

if freed from much of the inner stress that other babies have. They seem to worry less, are extremely cuddly, love to be held, and melt and mold into his parents' arms. Because of the special medical and emotional needs of your baby, you will periodically feel that you are giving, giving, giving, until you have no more to give. A fact of parenting handicapped babies that is not really appreciated is what your baby will give back to you. In my experience, parents who have developed a special type of parenting in harmony with the special needs of their child have developed an incredible sensitivity concerning their baby in particular and life in general. Your baby will help bring out a sensitive and nurturing nature in you that will carry over into all aspects of your life. This is especially true if there are older siblings. Parenting a special baby is a family affair. I have seen many instances where older children have mellowed out their egocentric and selfish natures and become very giving, nurturing, sensitive, and caring children. It is as if this special baby has helped the older children develop lifelong nurturing qualities.

Parenting a handicapped baby often causes marital stress. Because a high-need baby often elicits a high level of giving from his mother, I have seen instances when mothers totally focus on the special needs of the baby and withdraw from other social contacts and the needs of other members of the family. It is natural for a mother to feel, "My baby needs me so much, but my husband is a big boy and can take care of himself." In order for you to meet the incessant needs of a handicapped child, you will need the support of all the family members, especially your spouse. Don't neglect him or shut him out at this crucial time.

291. *We are expecting twins soon. Any survival tips?*

A family blessed with twins has twice the fun and twice the fatigue. Here are some suggestions:

1. Be prepared. The Mother of Twins Club is an excellent resource for helping you with your twins. (For information on your nearest M.O.T. Club contact: National Organization of Mothers of Twins Clubs, 5402 Amberwood Lane, Rockville, MD 20853, (301) 460-9108

2. Right after birth, instead of putting babies in separate bassinets in the hospital, most twins are quieter if placed side by side or face to face in the same bassinet. After all, they have been womb mates for nine months. Over the next few months you can determine whether they sleep best in the same or in separate beds.

3. Get help. Although twins are a beautiful blessing, they can also overtax the reserves of most parents. Get help for the household duties, especially for the first few months. Household help is not a luxury for parents of twins, it is a necessity. The best gifts well-meaning friends can give to parents of twins are housekeeping help, care of other siblings, and an occasional dinner.

4. Father involvement is not an option, it is a must. Well-defined mother–father roles are not as clear-cut with twins. As one father of twins in our practice put it, "Our babies have two mothers; she's the milk mother and I'm the everything-else mother. We're both on twenty-four-hour duty." A sense of humor will help you survive.

5. Be organized. Parenting twins demands resourcefulness and organization. Devise shortcuts in food preparation, feeding your twins, dressing, bathing, shopping, and household management. Parents of twins can give you valuable advice in these areas.

6. You are parenting individuals, not twins. Refer to them as "Mary and Bobby" rather than "the twins." There are no absolute do's or dont's about treating twins as individuals. As they grow older, you will find that they may tend to play both ends. They like both the special feeling of being twins and the special feeling of being individuals. One day they may want to dress alike; the next day they may want to dress very differently. Go

with the flow and respect their wishes when they want to be twins and when they want to be individuals.

The fatigue of the early years of parenting twins is usually rewarded in the later years when you witness the emergence of a very special relationship. A valuable information and support resource is the Mother of Twins Club in your area. The club can tell you how to order a helpful newsletter, "Double Talk."

292. *Our baby is one-year-old and I am returning to full-time work. I need some tips in selecting a day-care center.*

In selecting day care for your child, keep in mind that you are searching for substitute parents—in other words, for care givers who share your values. Here are some suggestions:

1. Visit the prospective day-care center and draw your own conclusions about whether the needs of your child will be met in that particular environment.
2. What is the ratio of care givers to children? One care giver can usually care for the needs of no more than four infants.
3. What are the credentials of the staff? Is the staff genuinely sensitive to the needs of babies? A leading question you can ask is: "What will you do when my baby cries?" You are looking for a comforting and responsive answer such as "I will try to find out why she is crying and do my best to comfort her." Beware of answers like "It's good for babies to cry sometimes; you don't want to spoil her by picking her up all the time." What are their methods of discipline? Does the staff have special training in cognitive development and stimulation of children at various stages? Most important, are the staff truly nurturing people?

   Examine the personality of the person who will be caring for your child. Watch her in action. Is she sensitive to the child as a person? Does she enjoy eye-to-eye contact with your child? Does she touch her often? Does she talk to her in a way that shows she really cares what she feels? Language (visual, tactile, and vocal) is a powerful communication tool that conveys caring. Is she flexible? Is she able to adapt to the everchanging moods of some toddlers? Does she have a genuine sense of humor, which is a must in order to cope with toddlers? Watch how the children relate to the care giver. If a child has that certain sparkle in her eye as she relates to her care giver, you can be sure that the child is comfortable with her. Small children are often the best critics of their own care.

4. Is the philosophy of the center designed to strengthen the family unit and supplement home care rather than replace it?

5. Are the facilities clean? Is the equipment safe and appropriate for various age groups? Unfortunately, the same economic constraints that compel mothers to work also prevent some day-care centers from hiring the quantity and quality of staff and equipment necessary to provide a first-rate facility. In addition to day-care centers, you may also wish to look into the alternative of leaving your one-year-old in the care of another mother in her own home or your home. Many very nurturing mothers prefer to stay at home with their child in the early years, but need to supplement their income by giving day care in their own homes to one or two children in addition to their own.

293. *We are a happy family with six children. They have been a blessing to us, but we occasionally get flack from well-meaning friends about the world already being over-populated. How can we deal with these remarks?*

Diplomatically. Some people are still caught up with the idea of 2.2 children (the national average), as if exceeding it violates some biological law! Here's an answer given by a friend of ours in defending her position on how proud she is to have reared five well-disciplined children: "The world needs my children." That says it all!

294. *I am soon marrying a widower with three children, ages three, seven, and thirteen. I have never had children of my own and I'm apprehensive about my new role. Help!*

There are many individual concerns which underlie stepparenting and "blended families." Here are some general suggestions: You probably have an overwhelming desire to be accepted by your husband's children. However, you should remember that instant intimacy is not always possible when a stepparent enters the family. Expect a gradual warm-up period as the children attempt to sort out just what role you are going to have with them and they with you. Try not to become overly zealous as their "mother" right away. They may need you to be a friend to them first of all. Start by being a fun person to be around and gradually ease into the role of mother once you build up their trust. This is especially true with teenagers.

Anticipate some initial awkwardness in disciplining the children. Authority must be first based on trust, and that is usually built up over a period of many years by the biological parent. It is important for your husband to pave the way for your role as an authority figure and disciplinarian, but again, gradual build-up is the key. Children are exquisitely sensitive to the way in which you treat their father. Demonstrating that a loving and caring relationship exists between you and your new husband should win you points with the children.

Children have a remarkable sense of honesty and fairness. Be honest with them, especially the older children. If you are uncertain about your role in a given situation, talk it over with them. Don't try to fake it, for children are keenly perceptive when a person is not genuine. Every stepmother cannot be a Julie Andrews in *The Sound of Music*. Even she had to weather the initiation of frogs in her pocket and pine cones on her chair seat. Once the children realized that they really did need her and she was a person who could be trusted and fun to be with, the new family blended together.

295. *I am recently coping with the role of a single parent following a nasty divorce. I have custody of our two preschool children, but I am having trouble with discipline. Can you give me some advice?*

The custodial parent must continue household routines and enforce family discipline. Depending on the previous family involvement by the husband, many mothers find coping by themselves extremely difficult. Following a divorce, household routines often become disorganized and discipline is relaxed. At a time when organization and consistent discipline are needed, your capacity to parent the whole household diminishes because you are trying to reorganize yourself. Try the following strategies to cope with this dilemma:

1. Children do not adapt well to too many changes too fast. If changes (e.g., different house, school, city) are necessary, attempt these gradually and with preparation. Family life must go on and obviously some changes are necessary. As your children get a bit older they will have to accept some increased responsibility. This is a nonnegotiable fact of single-parent family life. Who will now do what can be negotiated at a family council, when you call the children together and make a list of the new responsibilities to be shared and let each child have a say in choosing his contribution. Forcing too many responsibilities on your children at this vulnerable time may make them rebel and further resent the divorce. Organization in the household makes the children's total adjustment and your discipline much easier to deal with.

3. Single parents have to run a tight ship. Remember, discipline also implies emotional support. If you increase both your expectations of your children and your methods of conveying your love to them, they will most likely respect the changes in discipline.

4. Following a divorce or death, a single parent frequently moves back to the town of the grandparents. They can provide valuable support, both for the parent, who needs love and companionship, and for the children, who may

need the love and care only a blood relative can offer. Your children may gravitate to the grandfather as a father figure, which is usually healthy behavior. Single-parent organizations and religious groups may also provide you with social contacts and valuable support.

5. You cannot be both a mother and father to your children. This cliché is unrealistic. If you are a good mother, be a good mother; if you are a good father, continue to be a good father. Many single mothers are understandably concerned about providing male role models in their children's lives. Mothers are not expected to become football players and fishermen overnight. You *can* provide opportunities for your children to meet males who will act as role models at school, clubs, religious and sports events. Appreciate that a male role model is not a substitute for a continued father–child relationship. The primary goal in parenting your child through a divorce is to preserve his sense of security within the divided family.

Most preschool children of divorce experience the following types of behaviors. Because many preschool children do not verbalize their feelings, they may show regressive behavior. This results from a sense of loss and insecurity, and may consist of thumb sucking, masturbation, mood swings, and sleep disturbances (caused by a fear of waking up and finding mommy gone too). Children may also regress in developmental progress, such as toilet training. The preschool child may cling to the custodial parent for fear of losing that parent too. He may crave attention and not let you out of his sight. He may also feel that he is to blame for daddy's departure. The child's energy demands and behavioral changes put an added strain on you as a custodial parent at the same time that you are struggling with your own adjustment. If possible, delay any sudden changes in your parent–child relationship, such as a return to work or school, for a few months. Your preschool child may be too young to understand your needs and may interpret your departures as abandonment. Try to accept his desire to sleep with you and go with you wherever you go. Let him be near you as often as possible.

296. *My wife and I are getting a divorce. I really love my five-year-old and want her to feel she always will have me as her father. What should I do?*

1. Tell your child as soon as the decision to separate is final. This allows her some time for adjustment between the initial shock and actual departure of one parent from the home. Telling your child early allows time for continued questions and dialogue about a divorce, and enables both parents to support the child's adjustment anxieties.
2. Tell your child what divorce actually means in your situation. She should understand that you will no longer live in the house if your wife has custodial care, and she needs to know where you will be living.
3. Define exactly what your role will be in your child's care. She is bound to feel that not only is "mommy losing daddy" but she is "losing daddy" too. You must impress upon her that she has not lost her father. She needs to understand how your relationship will continue, where you will live, how often she will see you, etc. Defining your role exactly may, of course, be difficult if you have not answered this question yet yourself.
4. Tell your child the reason for the divorce if possible, in language and detail appropriate to her age and level of understanding. Details of marital infidelity should be withheld, since they serve no useful purpose. The rationalization that divorce is common these days has no meaning to a child. She is concerned about her own family and not general social customs. It is extremely important that your child feels reassured that she is not the cause of the divorce.
5. Tell your child how often you plan to visit. Ideally, visiting a young child should be like her feeding schedule—small, frequent visits on an as-needed basis.
6. As your child gets older, consult with her to work out a

visiting arrangement that respects her busy schedule. Scheduled visiting rights are somewhat artificial, especially for older children. Your child may have some important activity and be ambivalent about spending a weekend with dad. Perhaps an open visiting arrangement is more realistic for older children. For example, you could call up and say, "How would you like to go to dinner or a ball game tonight?" thus giving the child the option to spend time with you. Spending every weekend with dad is a situation far removed from the reality of family life and can be confusing to the child. These weekends may also be unrealistic because they often consist entirely of fun and games, which is totally different from the child's life at home. Occasional visits of a Disneyland daddy are fun for a child, but a steady diet is not a realistic way of life. These problems can be avoided during your time with your child if you as a non-custodial parent maintain a discipline similar to the one which prevails at home; otherwise, your child becomes confused and, worse, learns to play one parent against the other. Whatever your situation, continually reassure your child that you will always be her daddy.

297. *Still breastfeeding our eighteen-month-old child, I am soon divorcing my husband. My child is very attached to me and she breastfeeds once at night. My husband wants her to be with him every other weekend, and I feel she is not ready for that. We are currently having a legal battle over this. Help!*

Having been a consultant in several legal cases such as yours, I ask you to consider first what is best for your child and not for the parents in this case, and above all to resist the temptation to use your child against your husband. I have seen mothers who have used extended nursing as a tool to prolong attachment and keep the father from overnight visitation. If you genuinely feel that your child is not ready to wean and it would not be in her best interest to be separated from you for a day or two, let me give you some suggestions. Some very securely attached eighteen-month-olds are truly not ready for twenty-four- to forty-eight-hour separations from their mothers. It would be devastating to their emotional health and have a detrimental effect on the relationship between mother and child and father and child. It is a no-win situation for all three of you. A wise compromise is to offer more frequent visits but for shorter periods of time. Begin with a few hours several times a week, gradually allowing overnight visits as your child begins to wean. This requires some maturity from both you and the child's father in taking cues from the child as to how long a separation from her mother she can realistically be expected to tolerate. Don't use your child's needs to prevent her father from seeing her. A court cannot legislate time of weaning (although some have attempted to).

When the baby's father is not in agreement with your mothering style (i.e., sharing sleep, timing of the weaning process, etc.), he is, unfortunately, likely to attack these practices in court. If that is your case, you should send for the Legal Rights packet available from La Leche League International, P.O. Box 1209, Franklin Park, IL 60131-8209.

298. *We are expecting a new baby in a few months. How should we prepare our two-and-a-half-year-old to accept his new brother or sister?*

Begin introducing your child to "his" new baby during your pregnancy. Let him feel the baby move and encourage him to talk to the baby, saying things like "I'm your big brother and I'll help take care of you." Begin modeling (if you haven't already) a gentle touching atmosphere so that he learns that big people are gentle to little people. Show him picture books of the developing baby and prepare him for what new babies are really going to be like: New babies need to be nursed a lot, held a lot, touched softly and quietly, etc.

Most hospitals now encourage visits from siblings shortly

or immediately after the new baby's birth so that your child does not feel suddenly displaced from his mother. Many hospitals even offer new sibling classes as part of the preparation for childbirth class. During the early months after the birth you should emphasize the special things about your older child as much as possible: how you appreciate his help in taking care of the baby, how mommy and daddy love their older child as much as their new baby. A wise gift-bearing friend usually brings over a gift for the older sibling as well as for the baby. Let your child unwrap the baby gifts for you if he wants to and encourage him to "give" the presents to his baby. Some experts also feel a special gift from the newborn to the older child on the day of homecoming helps foster warm feelings.

Older children like to play with dolls like mommy "plays" with the new baby. If you have a baby carrier for your new baby, make a little scarf-like sling for your older child to carry his baby around in. Be prepared for mood swings. There will be days when your older child wants to be a big boy and days when he wants to be a baby also. Go with the flow. In essence, you want to convey to your older child the attitude that big people nurture little people. This modeling will carry over to the next generation when your child becomes a parent.

299. *We are considering getting our two-year-old a dog. Any suggestions on selecting the right pet?*

Pets provide companionship and enrich the life of a growing child. Like toys, pets provide enjoyment but also possible dangers to the child and inconveniences to parents. Animals that have been bred to be pets usually make the best companions. Wild animals exhibit unpredictable behavior in captivity and are difficult to care for since we know less about their nutritional, medical, and behavioral needs. Even exotic wild animals bred in captivity do not usually make good pets. Stick to the old reliable dog or cat. Select a breed which is known to be gentle with children, such as a Labra-

dor retriever. Avoid breeds which have high-strung person-
alities such as little "yappers" who often compensate for
their size with unpredictable and unpleasant behavior. Take
time in selecting the right dog and make a wise investment,
since the dog is likely to be part of the family for many
years.

To select a healthy pet, watch for obvious danger signs
such as discharge from the eyes, diarrhea, cough, patches
of missing hair, or skin problems. Let your child play with
the prospective pet for a while before selecting it. Be sure
your child and the pet get along and your child is not allergic. (Does she sneeze or wheeze after spending an hour or
two with the pet?) Do this before bringing the pet home.
Once it is part of the family, giving it up is very hard no
matter how allergic the child is to it. If you are uncertain
about the pet's health, ask a veterinarian to check over the
animal before you make a final decision.

300. *I'm concerned about child abuse. The other day I saw
my neighbor hit her two-year-old on the head for what
seemed to me to be a small show of childish irresponsibility
rather than real defiance. Her child seems very scared of
her and I wonder if this goes on all the time. She is my
friend. Should I mind my own business or intervene?*

This *is* your business. You have an obligation to the child
and the mother to offer help. The incident you witnessed
may be only the tip of the iceberg. There may be a lot of
stress going on in this family, and the mother, by hitting
her child, may be really saying, "I need help." Approach
your friend in love, showing that you care enough to con-
front her. Don't start off by being accusative and judg-
mental. Above all, don't accuse her of child abuse, but rather
ask her if she needs some help in discipline. I sense from
your question that you feel that this is not an isolated incident in which a mother lost her cool, but rather a habitual
pattern of beating, which is child abuse. You need to act on
your intuition. Encourage your friend to seek professional

help in this matter. If she refuses your help or professional counseling, you have an obligation to report your suspicions to the nearest child-abuse authorities, which you can do anonymously. Ignored child abuse usually leads to tragic consequences. Intervene now and you may save a life, a marriage, and hopefully a friendship.

APPENDIX

PARENTING RESOURCES

CHILDBIRTH EDUCATION ASSOCIATIONS

1. The International Childbirth Educational Association (ICEA).
   P.O. Box 20048
   Minneapolis, MN 55420
   (612) 854-8660
2. ASPO - Lamaze
   1411 K Street Northwest
   Washington, D.C. 20051
   (202) 783-7050
3. The American Academy of Husband-Coached Childbirth—the Bradley method.
   P.O. Box 5224
   Sherman Oaks, CA 91413
   (213) 788-6662
4. National Association of Parents and Professionals for Safe Alternatives in Childbirth (NAPSAC)

P.O. Box 267
Marble Hill, MO 63764
(314) 238-2010

BREASTFEEDING RESOURCES

1. La Leche League International
   P.O. Box 1209
   Franklin Park, IL 60131-8209
   1-800-LaLeche or (708) 455-7730
2. *Breastfeeding—Getting the Right Start*
   By Martha and William Sears
   This introductory manual for the new breastfeeding
   mother teaches a step-by-step photographic approach to
   proper positioning and latch-on techniques as well as
   overcoming the most common breastfeeding problems. It
   is available from Creative Parenting Resources, P.O. Box
   7238, Capistrano Beach, CA 92624.
3. International Lactation Consultant Association (ILCA)
   P.O. Box 4031
   University of Virginia Station
   Charlottesville, VA 22903
   (704) 664-1054

RESOURCES FOR DOWN'S SYNDROME AND OTHER DEVELOPMENTALLY DELAYED CHILDREN

1. Handicapped Children's Early Education Program
   Office of Special Education (OSE)
   U.S. Department of Education
   Switzer Building, Room 4605
   400 Maryland Avenue SW
   Washington, DC 20202
   (202) 429-7800
2. National Association for Down's Syndrome
   P.O. Box 4542
   Oakbrook, IL 60521
   (312) 325-9112

3. Down Syndrome Congress
   1640 West Roosevelt Road
   Chicago, IL 60608
4. National Down Syndrome Society
   130 Fifth Avenue
   New York, NY 10011
   1-800-221-4602

RESOURCES FOR CHILD SPACING AND NATURAL FAMILY PLANNING

1. Kippley, S. *Breastfeeding and Natural Child Spacing.* New York: Penguin Books, 1974.

COUPLE-TO-COUPLE LEAGUE

P.O. Box 111184
Cincinnati, OH 45211

RESOURCES FOR SUDDEN INFANT DEATH SYNDROME (SIDS)

National Sudden Infant Death Foundation
300 S. Michigan Avenue
Chicago, IL
(312) 663-0650

RESOURCES FOR CPR CLASSES

American Red Cross
Local Chapter
See local phone book

RESOURCE INFORMATION FOR INFANTS' AND CHILDREN'S FOOTWEAR

"The Ten Most Asked Questions About Babies' Feet," by William Sears, M.D. This informative booklet answers most

of the questions parents have about choosing the right shoes for their infant and child; available from:
Stride-Rite Footwear, Inc.
5 Cambridge Center
Cambridge, MA 02142

MEDICAL RESOURCES

1. American Academy of Pediatrics
   P.O. Box 1034
   1801 Hinman Avenue
   Evanston IL 60201
   (312) 869-4255
2. American Medical Association
   535 North Dearborn Street
   Chicago, IL 60610
   (312) 751-6000

Acetaminophen Dosage

Doses should be administered 4 or 5 times daily—but not to exceed 5 doses in 24 hours.

Age Group	0-3 mos	4-11 mos	12-23 mos	2-3 yrs	4-5 yrs	6-8 yrs	9-10 yrs	11-12 yrs
Weight (lbs)	6-11	12-17	18-23	24-35	36-47	48-59	60-71	72-95
Dose of acetaminophen in milligrams (mg)	40	80	120	160	240	320	400	480
Drops (80 mg/0.8 ml) dropperfuls	½	1	1½	2	3	4	5	—
Elixir (160 mg/5 ml) tsp.	—	½	¾	1	1½	2	2½	3
Chewable tables (80 mg each)	—	—	1½	2	3	4	5	6
Suppositories (120 mg each)	One suppository/year of age 4 times/day							

SUGGESTED PARENTS' LIBRARY

Good, Julia Darnell and Joyce Good Reis. *A Special Kind of Parenting: Meeting the needs of Handicapped Children.* Franklin Park, Ill.: La Leche League, 1985.

Klaus, Marshall and John Kennel. *Parent-Infant Bonding.* St. Louis: C.V. Mosby, 1982.

Korte, Diana and Roberta Scaer. *A Good Birth, A Safe Birth.* New York: Bantam, 1989.

La Leche League International. *The Womanly Art of Breastfeeding.* New York: New American Library, 1983.

McClure, Vimala Schneider. *Infant Massage: A Handbook for Loving Parents.* New York: Bantam, 1989.

Montagu, Ashley. *Touching: The Human Significance of the Skin.* New York: Columbia Univ. Press, 1971.

Sears, Martha. *Breastfeeding: Getting the Right Start.* Capistrano Beach, Cal.: Creative Parenting Resources, 1990.

SUGGESTED MAGAZINES

Baby Talk, 636 Avenue of the Americas, New York, NY 10011.

Baby on the Way, also published by *Baby Talk* magazine.

Index

ABC rooms, 2
Abdominal pain, 140, 196,
    205–06
Accident prevention, 187–97,
    222–23
Acetominophen, 54, 182, 195,
    198, 220, 282
Adopted baby, breastfeeding,
    52
Aggressiveness, 252
Airplane travel, 220
Allergies, 176–81. *See also* Food
    allergies
Alpha fetal protein test, 9
American Academy of Obstetri-
    cians and Gynecologists
    (ACOG), 6
American Academy of Pediat-
    rics, 15, 27, 137, 138, 140,
    141, 149, 192, 219
American Heart Association,
    138
Ammonia, 194
Amniocentesis, 9
Anemia, 141, 143, 148–49
Anesthetic, for circumcision, 16
Antibiotics
    and diarrhea, 185
    to prevent ear infection, 180–
        81

    safety of, 185–86
Antibodies, 73
Apgar, Dr. Virginia, 18
Apgar score, 18
Apple juice, 136
Areola, 60
Artificial coloring, 250
Ask About Your Baby (radio
    program), ix
Aspirin, 54, 182, 195, 198
Attachment parenting, x, 62,
    225–26, 241–42, 255–56
Attention
    deficit disorder (ADD), 250
    holding baby's, 162–64
Avocados, 137, 150

Baby
    accidents, 189–97, 222–23
    behavior problems, 225–41
    birthing and first days, 1–44
    breastfeeding, 45–86
    and family stress, 261–78
    fathering, 154–74
        feeding and nutrition, 126–
            52
    illnesses, 176–87
    preventive medicine, 197–224
    sleep problems, 85–125

285